YOGA ASANAS

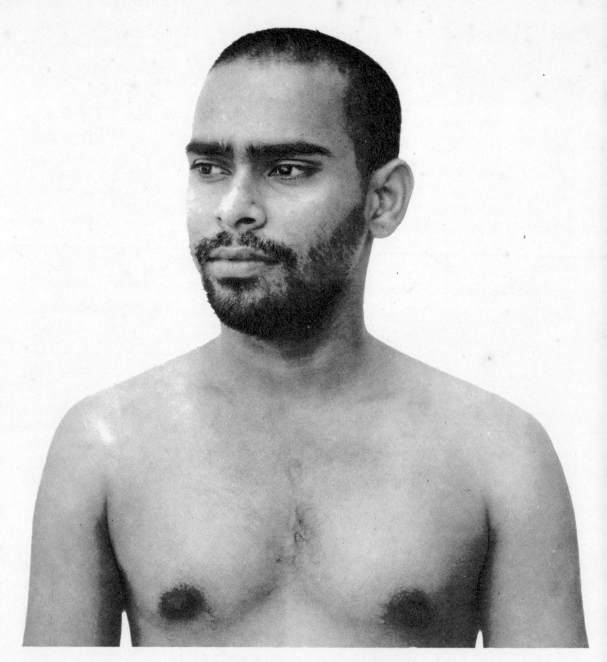

SWAMI-VISHNOUDEVANANDA

YOGA ASANAS

A NATURAL METHOD OF PHYSICAL AND MENTAL TRAINING

by

LOUIS FRÉDÉRIC

INTRODUCTION AND POSES
by

SWAMI-VISHNOUDEVANANDA

PROFESSOR OF HATHA YOGA AT THE
FOREST UNIVERSITY
RISHIKESH, HIMALAYAS

PHOTOGRAPHS BY LOUIS FRÉDÉRIC

TRANSLATED FROM THE FRENCH
by
GEOFFREY A. DUDLEY, B.A.

THORSONS PUBLISHERS LTD.
91 St. Martin's Lane, London, W.C.2

Original French Edition published 1956
by
EDITIONS J. OLIVEN, Paris

First English Edition 1959

© *Thorsons Publishers Ltd. 1959*

MADE AND PRINTED IN GREAT BRITAIN BY
MORRISON AND GIBB LIMITED, LONDON AND EDINBURGH

FOREWORD

YOGA is a Hindu science of bodily and mental control. It is one of the six classic philosophical systems of India. A disciple of this ancient teaching is called a Yogi. He is an adept who has attained a spiritual illumination.

The traditional founder of Yoga is Patanjali, who is believed to have lived about the third century B.C., and whose *Yogasutra* is the oldest text in the literature.

The name of this science is Sanskrit, meaning "union"; and Yoga aims at the union of the individual spirit with the Universal Spirit. In the West this is sometimes spoken of as "cosmic consciousness"; in Yoga it is known as *samadhi*. *Samadhi* is a state of profound meditation which cannot be described in words, but only experienced by the truly enlightened adept.

The attainment of cosmic consciousness is the main object of Yoga, but it also has less exalted aims, with which this book is largely concerned. It aims to free man from pain arising from his own infirmities and wrong conduct and from his relations with other living things and external Nature.

This goal is accomplished in eight stages, of which union with the Universal Soul is the culmination. The first two stages are concerned with self-control and self-culture. Yoga counsels the practice of moral virtues, such as avoidance of injury to others, truthfulness, forgiveness, compassion, sincerity and so on. It also prescribes rules of inner control, such as contentment, charity, modesty and sacrifice. These are matters of conduct and character which are not unique to Yoga, but to which other systems of physical and mental training and discipline can also lay claim.

What is unique to Yoga is the emphasis it places on correct postures (asanas) combined with breath-control. These are the third and fourth steps, and they form the subject-matter of *Yoga Asanas*. Their mastery is essential to the later stages, with which, however, we are not directly concerned here.

The asanas, posed by Swami-Vishnoudevananda and described and photographed by Louis Frédéric, constitute a system of physical culture which confers specific health benefits.

The author points out that the practice of the Yoga postures should be accompanied by correct breathing. Yoga gives to breathing an importance equal to that given to the other physical and mental aspects of the subject. Genuine Yogis are said to be able to accomplish amazing feats by breath-control. It is even claimed that psychic powers come during the course of development. Louis Frédéric, however, is chiefly concerned with the health benefits that follow from breath-control in conjunction with the asanas and relaxation.

Pursuing the tradition of other pioneer investigators, the author of this book studied the subject in India, where the photographs he presents were taken. At the well-known Forest University at Rishikesh he learned the Yoga asanas which are described and illustrated here for the benefit of the Western reader.

In introducing this translation of *Yoga Asanas*, the publishers are confident that the appeal that the work has already had for French-speaking readers will be equally as great for English-speaking ones, to whom it is now offered for the first time.

CONTENTS

LIST OF ILLUSTRATIONS

PREFACE

"AUM TAT SAT"

YOGA is a science which teaches how to awake our latent powers and hasten the process of human evolution. This technique was discovered by the ancient teachers of Yoga through the medium of intuition. According to what they say, the soul is enveloped by different vehicles and expressions of different degrees of density. The physical body is the lowest form of expression. These different vehicles manifest themselves according to different planes of consciousness, such as the physical plane, the astral plane, the mental plane, etc. The spirit is surrounded by five envelopes, physical, vital, mental, intellectual and divine. When man develops himself, his consciousness rises from the lower planes to the higher planes. As it attains the highest planes, man becomes more and more desirous of knowing his highest nature, and new possibilities and qualities come to him.

The lowest form of all the vehicles of the soul is the physical body, which is the grossest manifestation of man. The body is necessary to man's growth. It must be carefully looked after and trained so as to make it more perfect and bear the spirit to the loftiest goal. Everyone must try to make the body attain the highest degree of perfection possible, so that it may achieve its aim soundly and swiftly. Hatha Yoga teaches man the way to attain this stage.

We perceive all our worldly experiences through the body and mind. But the things which lie outside our conception are known only when the functions of the body, mind and senses are completely stopped. The highest experiences come man's way only when he is in complete accord with his true nature, with his soul. He realises then that Power and Energy are truly its nature. The mind and senses borrow their light from the soul, thus believing that they are the only causes of pleasure or pain, and man tries to fulfil his desires by making use of them.

Now the question arises of knowing how experiences can occur without the aid of the body nor of the mind. The answer is that in dreams the mind creates all objects in itself without any external contact with those objects. At the same time the whole process of dreaming is an absolute reality to the experimenter as long as he stays on the plane of dreaming. Let us now see what happens when man is plunged into a state of deep sleep. There the functions of the mind cease too. Man is in a state in which inner and outer experiences cannot affect him. He is neither troubled by anxiety nor concerned about the quest of pleasure because his mind is detached from everything. But, when he awakes, he knows that he has been in a deep sleep and is glad of the blessing it confers. It is clear that this satisfaction comes from the withdrawal of the mind.

So we have an idea of what can happen when body, mind and senses are brought to a state of quiescence by Yoga exercises. Experiences in the state of deep sleep and those arising from suspension of mental activity and breathing are, however, of different kinds. The man who awakens has acquired no knowledge nor the possibility of any, and is as ignorant as he was before going to sleep. But a man returning from the superconscious state produced by the cessation of mental activity and breathing possesses extraordinary attainments due to direct contact with the soul.

Yoga is thus a method in which modifications of mind, body and senses and breathing are first controlled, then stilled. When the latter state is attained, the real nature of the mind is awakened. It is thus a tendency towards a positive stage of pure consciousness through the cessation of all thinking and the absorption of the mind and vital breath.

In accordance with the different mental temperaments, Yoga has been divided into four different paths: Karma Yoga for active temperaments, Bhakti Yoga for emotional temperaments, and Raja and Jnana Yoga for intellectual temperaments. Raja Yoga includes three main branches: Mantra Yoga, Laya Yoga and Hatha Yoga.

The Yoga asanas described in this book are taken from Hatha Yoga. This gives preference to the physical body, which is the existence and the activity of the living being. Purity of the mind is not possible without purity of the body in which it functions and by which it is affected. The consecutive steps of Hatha Yoga are: concentration, meditation and the state of superconsciousness.

The philosophy and aims of Yoga are thus given very briefly.

In this small book Mr. Louis Frédéric has taken pains to collect the various asanas which Westerners can practise without danger and has given their uses. It is possible to achieve a very high degree of health and strength by practising the asanas and breath control.

The asanas are natural movements of the limbs and joints which allow the blood to circulate freely to every organ of the body. A person who is weak and in poor health is known to become irritable. In the same way, when the body is sick, one's mind cannot concentrate even on the most everyday tasks. That proves that the body influences the mind. When a person is constipated, the nervous system is affected and that may lead to mental depression. Science has proved the importance of the endocrine glands. If the secretion of these glands is deficient, the body may age prematurely and even die.

Yoga Asanas bring those who practise them a harmonious development of the whole body. While physical exercises pay special attention to the external muscles, asanas get right to the heart of the various organs by contractions and twists of the muscles and joints.

By means of the photos of the asanas taken by Mr. Louis Frédéric you will be able to understand how the human body can be trained to practise all these exercises. Constant and regular endeavours will assure you of success. You will also be able to discover from the poses what muscles and joints are brought into play and what internal organs are involved in the contractions. Some knowledge of anatomy and physiology will be of great value to the user. The endocrine glands play an important part in the economy of human nature and it is essential to strengthen them. The thyroid gland is one of the most important and is toned up by the described exercises. The other glands, such as the adrenals, the pituitary and the pineal, are also toned up and kept in good shape. Stagnation of blood in the arteries and veins is prevented and blood circulates freely in the entire body. Most Yoga postures are excellent for the spine, the most important structure of the body. Almost all the asanas give direct or indirect bends and twists to the spinal column. It is essential to have a lithe and supple body to stay young and full of vigour.

We have seen the difference between a young man and an old man. Suppleness disappears with age. Thanks to Yoga Asanas you can keep this suppleness and the joints remain flexible even in old age. The arteries do not harden. After the asanas and control of the breath the body receives extra energy and can perform more work than was possible to it before. Yoga also teaches how to rest the muscles and nerves by the technique of relaxation. Thus it proves to be a perfect system of physical culture and everybody, young or old, boy or girl, ought to know and practise these asanas. They are not only physical exercises as in other systems, for we have seen that they serve to control body and mind and achieve mental concentration. In this book only the asanas and breath control are indicated which form a complete system of training for mind and body.

This book will be of great use to Westerners who have not yet studied the science of Yoga and desire to make a start in it.

AUM TAT SAT

SWAMI-VISHNOUDEVANANDA

Rishikesh, 1955.

14

GENERAL REMARKS AND PRESENTATION
OF THE METHOD

CHAPTER I

FROM remotest times, long before the Greeks, who first systematised the different exercises which the human body is capable of carrying out, physical training has appealed to the young of every country. They have sought in it a break from the monotony of life and a means of education enabling them the better to face the rigours of existence and social competition, or even to conquer Nature the more easily with increased chances of success.

Several methods have been devised in turn without any giving full satisfaction. This is due to several reasons. In fact, individual sport seldom had the support of a naturally turbulent youth. It lacks the competition proper to other kinds of sport and the rivalry due to the differences in physical capabilities which can be observed in any group of human beings. Mainly composed of very simple movements, such individual exercises are monotonous enough to deter the keenest enthusiast. They bring him appreciable rewards only after very long and tedious efforts. They bring into play only the muscles and all they need is strength and suppleness. Such movements affect neither the circulation of the blood nor the correct functioning of the internal organs, still less the nerve currents which govern most of the functions of our body. They are seldom movements of relaxation, but rather exercises which tend to harden and inflate just the muscles. Very often this is to the detriment of other parts or organs of our body, which, compressed by over-inflated muscles and exhausted by the immense outlay of energy which they demand, cannot develop and work normally.

So-called eurhythmics, which are groups of individual movements, Swedish drill and so on have never yet cured or even prevented the various ills to which flesh is heir. The least illness can lay low the strongest athlete, and it is well known that the stronger a man is and the more muscles he has, the more is he liable to the various afflictions which beset the path of human life. The slightest bout of constipation upsets the whole life of a normally constituted person.

Team games themselves seek above all to achieve an aim, which is almost always victory for one's own side, and are little concerned with the physiological balance of the body. They especially develop in the one who plays them an *esprit de corps* and an understanding between human beings which is limited to an extremely small social group—the team.

Then there are competitive games, which have always been very popular and which, unfortunately, are the worst form of development that can be imagined. From the physical point of view they develop in those who play them only the part of the body used in a particular sport. For example, a tennis player who is right-handed may quite well possess a very weak left arm. A racing cyclist may have highly developed nerves and muscles of the legs, but, on the other hand, a round back and little lung capacity. Running, boxing, wrestling, jumping, etc., are in fact designed to enhance the possibilities of the human body in a restricted field and a limited time. Boxing has never prevented the boxer from having stomach disorders and has never yet developed his mental faculties. I have never heard speak of a racing cyclist who reached the age of forty still in possession of all his faculties. At that age he is considered as "finished." This kind of competition, in which the individual has the intense desire to beat his rival, if only by a few tenths of a second, has lost all its meaning as physical culture. It wears out the body of the participant rather than renews it or, more simply, even preserves it.

Besides, to keep in form a champion is tied to a physical and dietary régime which, however excellent for the muscles, is most of the time disastrous for the balance of his mental and physical health.

Several methods have so far been suggested to overcome these drawbacks. Hebertism, a kind of liaison between man and Nature, getting the human body used to overcoming a certain category of natural obstacles, develops especially qualities of speed, judgment and balance. These are very useful, it is true, but they are not compensated by any invigoration of the internal organs of the body. Unarmed combat and Judo, violent sports of attack and defence, are intended to develop initiative, courage and balance rather than strength itself. They are sports based on the rational use of the laws of gravitation and inertia. They imply intensive exercises aimed at conscious automatism, and develop in those who are adepts in them remarkable suppleness and stability as well as excellent moral qualities. These are sports complete in themselves. But they are little concerned with the human body's resistance to disease.

We might call swimming the most perfect of sports in the sense that it constitutes a complete physical exercise. It makes for harmonious development of the muscles and certain internal organs such as the lungs, the spinal column and the abdominal walls. But it is an exercise which is practised in an unusual element, and so even certain vital functions such as breathing through the skin are blocked. This leads in the long run to more or less serious disorders of the circulation and nervous system. Besides, those who go in for professional swimming rapidly burn up their reserves and cannot practise for long.

In short, we can easily take note that most sports pursued to-day do as much harm as good. We don't claim here to replace them completely; we simply explain a scientific method of natural gymnastics which gives the human body very great resistance to different diseases, and which could with advantage be used by those who practise other sports to make up for what they lack.

What, then, must a method of physical culture consist of to be ideal?

The aims sought by all those who try to develop to the maximum the latent possibilities of the human body are many:

1. To possess enough physical and muscular strength to be able to fill an honourable place in society and solve the many problems set by the opposition of Nature.

2. To keep a youthful body as long as possible.

3. To give the human body the greatest resistance to the various afflictions which can destroy or reduce it.

4. To cure such afflictions if we already have them and delay the approach of death.

5. To acquire mental health and a mind free from fears and inhibitions due to being born in a society ruled by laws, taboos and social conventions.

All that is what we seek and all that is what we can win at the cost of some effort by the regular practice of a simple individual physical training—that of the asanas.

This method, otherwise known under the name of Hatha Yoga, was described for the first time in India by Patanjali for a religious purpose; then constantly revised, it has now reached such a perfection that it fulfils all the requirements of an ideal method of physical culture.

These asanas and exercises, difficult as they may seem, can yet be performed by everyone with, of course, a little practice and goodwill.

We have graded them in three stages or degrees, the order of which it would be definitely **unwise** to want to change.

The beginner must start at the beginning, even if he feels that he can accomplish certain of the exercises of a higher degree. Only after doing all the exercises of the first degree for a set time will he then be able to pass on with advantage and no risk to the higher stage. These exercises are not, as some seem to think, feats reserved for fakirs or experts. They are exercises to regenerate, invigorate and regulate the working of the muscles, viscera, glands, blood circulation and the nervous and lymphatic systems. They are not exercises to be performed anyhow, anywhere or at any time.

"Asana" in Sanskrit means literally "posture." It is, in fact, a science of the positions which the body can take in combination with breathing. This is very important. Any sportsman will tell you that the breath and its control and training are the guarantee of success. The mastery of breath is the essential condition without which none of the asanas described can bring lasting rewards. On the contrary, a wrong use of breathing and asanas can be dangerous, producing effects opposite to those counted on. A correct dose of medicine cures; a weak dose is ineffective; a concentrated dose can cause serious complications and even prove fatal. This is the greatest danger threatening anyone who wants to practise the asanas. To guard against it we have tried to note as carefully as possible for each posture the right way to breathe.

As a general rule, **never use force**. Nature is there to resist us. We must change her, but never treat her rough. If we do she will have her revenge. Little by little, with an unfailing will, even the hardest exercises will make you smile.

Allied to the asanas and breathing there are the exercises of stillness, that is to say, holding a posture for a certain length of time. This stillness, even for the simplest asanas, is very difficult to acquire. It requires a perfect mastery of the body and mind, and for that it must be carried out without the least twitching or stiffening of the muscles. It must be restful, never tiring.

As soon as you experience any fatigue or inconvenience, stop absolutely. You are quite free to start again a few hours later. There is no need to hurry. Let your own nature be your guide. There is no call for force, but for comfort. Only the latter is of any value.

Every morning, when you wake, drink a large glass of pure water: it is normal to wash inside as well as out.

Abstain from alcohol. Drink wine with your meals if you are used to it, but do away with aperitifs.

Don't smoke too much. Try not to smoke for at least two hours before your exercises.

Avoid excesses of any kind. Eat in moderation, especially green vegetables, fruit and dairy products. Not too many eggs, too much coffee or pork. Avoid sauces which are heavy to digest.

Every quest of perfection demands from the seeker a certain measure of will and self-denial. The ideal would, of course, be not to smoke at all, to drink neither wine nor spirits, and to follow a strictly vegetarian diet. But we know from experience that that is not possible except for very few people living in special circumstances. The average European, tied to his daily job and a more or less anxious life, cannot be satisfied with too frugal a régime. Enticed on all sides by pleasures to which he has been used for years and years, he cannot give them up without expending energy and will-power which would after all do him more harm than good. Here, too, let well alone. Common sense favours always trying to **strike the happy medium**. So let everyone do his best and try to profit to the utmost by the teachings which we are going to try to expound here.

The human body has a great many possibilities which, thousands of years ago, were much wider than those we possess now. In prehistoric times man was much closer to the animals, and we all know that they are much superior to us in most physical respects. We have quite simply degenerated and suffer from a lack of adaptation to the natural conditions which were those of the dawn of human life. These exercises, then, have as their main aim to restore to man the essence of the faculties which he has lost and enable him to recover in the highest degree the possibilities which his ancestors used to possess. In carrying out the various asanas which we are going to describe, the novice will not be opposing Nature but rather helping her to give him back the strength and vitality which are no longer his.

This course (for we can consider that this book is one) will thus be divided into six parts:

1. Exercises for controlling and regulating the breath.

2. Relaxation or the science of complete rest.

3. Combined movement or Salute to the Sun.

4. Asanas or postures of stillness, divided into three degrees.

5. Exercise for strengthening the abdominal organs (Group 30).

6. Specimen training chart.

The asanas proper are divided into thirty groups totalling seventy-eight different positions of increasing difficulty. We hope that the pupil will observe the advice we have given and we wish him the best of results. May he become stronger, spiritually, mentally and physically, and conquer disease, and we shall have achieved our aim.

TECHNIQUE OF CONTROLLED BREATHING

CHAPTER II

BREATHING is natural to man from birth. No one has taught him and he will never learn in the course of his life. He thinks he knows how to breathe. In reality breathing is to him an innate endowment like that of seeing, hearing or eating. But he does not know how to breathe. He lives by virtue of breathing automatically, and in general that is enough for him. It is curious to note that this, the most important fact of human life, has remained in the natural state, and that man has so rarely been concerned with studying or utilising it. For breathing is a science, the science of living, and of living in good health. All the sources of human energy lie in the few cubic inches of air inhaled each second. The 21,600 breaths taken each day represent over 800 cubic feet of air transformed in those factories which are models of regular functioning—the lungs. These simple figures amply prove how important it is to give them some attention.

The quantity and quality of the air we breathe and the rhythm at which it is taken in and changed into vital energy control the level of our mental and physical health as well as the length of our life. The more rapidly and shallowly a person breathes, the shorter his life. On the other hand, the slower and deeper his breaths, the greater his chances of living a long time. A butterfly, which lives at a very rapid rhythm, survives only a few hours; a tree, which breathes much more slowly, can live for hundreds of years.

The normal span of a man's life ought to be 120 years if we consider the rhythm at which he breathes while resting. Why has this prolongation never been achieved? Irregularity in human activity is the main reason for it. In fact, the rate of breathing in a man can vary from ten to forty respirations a minute according to whether he is sleeping or performing strenuous work. These, then, are the outside influences which condition the rate and volume of our breathing without our will having the least to do with it. From this point of view we live like machines. If we wish to improve in health and length of life, the thing is not to squander at random this stored-up energy but to exercise the maximum control over it.

It is impossible for us to control the breathing of the skin, this being a phenomenon independent of our will, as are the sugar-producing functions of the liver or the internal secretions. We can neither speed it up nor slow it down, and only outside influences can affect its working and change it to suit them. On the other hand, only the energy which we store up **via** the nostrils and expel once it is used by the same passages can be controlled, intensified or even completely stopped, independently of outside circumstances, by the sole exercise of our will. The latter, then, is the breathing which we ought to control and study.

The first thing is to **realise** that we breathe. Let us try. Sit down quietly, then take a deep breath. Retain the air for a few seconds, and breathe out so as to expel all the air in your lungs. Do this several times running as you try to concentrate your thought on the air going in through the nostrils, passing at the back of the nose and throat, down the windpipe, filling the lungs, pushing out the abdominal organs as it presses down the diaphragm, expanding the rib cage, then, like a bellows, making the return journey until it finally mixes with the air outside again. This simple little exercise will give you an idea of the importance of the vital breath. You will realise perhaps for the first time the exact process of this exceptional phenomenon—the nourishment of life by the absorption of energy which seems to be external to it.

The control of breath will be achieved then by spending a few minutes each day in mastering it. More particularly one should carry out the physical exercises which we are about to describe, forcing the breathing to have a precise rhythm based on alternating and stopping at will. Breathing itself consists of three phases: breathing in, holding the breath (the rib cage being full or empty), and breathing out. The best rhythm to adopt is in the following proportions:

Breathing in: 1.

Holding the breath: 4.

Breathing out: 2.

Pause: 4.

Contrary to currently expressed opinion, breathing out should be **always twice as long** as breathing in.

Now we will give you the following exercises:

EXERCISE 1

Sit in a comfortable position, in a chair or on the ground on a cushion, so that the spinal column and the nape of the neck are upright in a straight line. After eliminating from your mind everything that could distract it from the subject in hand, start by breathing slowly as you count in seconds, first breathing in for two seconds, then holding the breath for eight seconds, and breathing out for four seconds. Gradually increase the time, that is to say, three seconds, twelve seconds, six seconds, then four seconds, sixteen seconds, eight seconds, until your maximum possible slowness is reached. If you can hold your breath while your lungs are empty for as long as you hold it with them full, that will be better still. This, however, although recommended, is not compulsory.

Practise the above exercise for two minutes to start with, breathing through both nostrils together. Gradually increase the timing. Break off after ten minutes and practise the second exercise:

EXERCISE 2

Sit in the same position, or in any of the positions described in the diamond, hero, lotus asanas, etc. Keep the same rhythm of breathing, drawing in the air through each nostril alternately and expelling the breath through the other nostril. For example, you inhale for two seconds through the left nostril, hold the breath for eight seconds, and expel the air through the right nostril for four seconds. Keep the lungs empty for a moment or two, then inhale through the right nostril for two seconds, hold the breath for eight seconds and expel through the left nostril for four seconds. Then continue the same process, breathing in again through the left nostril, and so on.

To do it more easily, the fingers should be used to close the nostrils, at least to begin with. After a certain period of training it will be possible for you to breathe through one or other of the nostrils without having recourse to the fingers. The most comfortable position, which greatly assists concentration of the mind on the breath, is as follows:

Put the first and second fingers in the centre of the forehead between the eyebrows, then make use of the ring finger and thumb to stop each nostril alternately.

EXERCISE 3

Try to breathe as rapidly and deeply as you can through one nostril only. Keep the same time for breathing in and out, holding the breath only when the lungs are empty, not when they are full. But **never practise this exercise at the start** of your training without having previously done one of the first two for a few minutes at least.

Always finish the exercises, no matter how long they take and what kind they are, with the first one described above.

These three types of breathing lead to considerable changes in the person who practises them for a certain time. Those who consider themselves overweight will find them a radical means of slimming without risk. The voice becomes deeper, softer and sweeter, the lungs develop, the blood is purified, the appetite is keener, the burden of fatigue is lifted from the mind, and the brain faculties and memory are strengthened.

The third exercise particularly stimulates the digestive juices and prevents the body from feeling cold. It is especially recommended for querulous characters and all those who suffer from stomach and liver disorders and asthma.

In conjunction with the asanas, breath-control will rid you of excessive fatigue and increase the effects of the asanas. Devote at least five minutes to exercises of this kind before and after practising the asanas. While you are carrying out the latter make sure that you stick to the advice on breathing. This is very important, for an asana practised with inadequate breathing may in the long run become harmful and even dangerous to health.

Little by little, as you regularly practise these exercises, you will come to do them instinctively whenever physical or mental fatigue makes itself felt. That will help you a great deal all your life.

PHYSICAL AND MENTAL RELAXATION

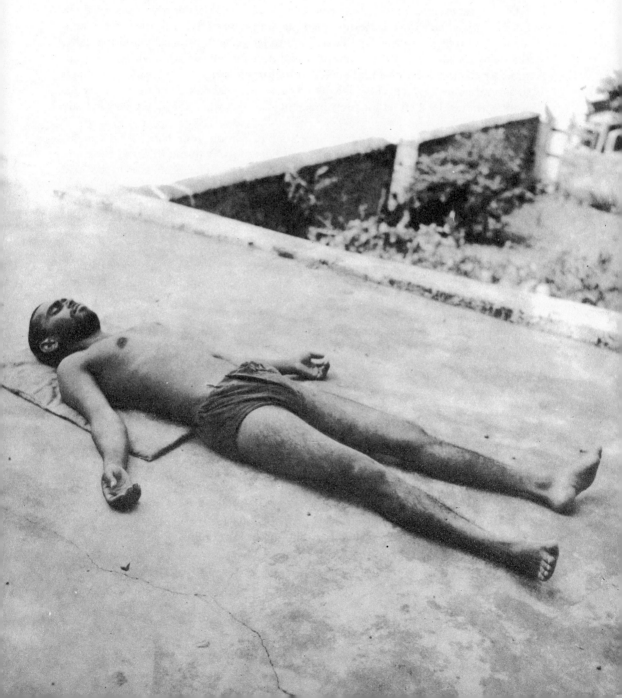

CHAPTER III

NO physical exercise or breathing can be of value if the person who practises them does not know how to rest. Resting does not simply mean lying down and thinking about the problems of the day. To relax is to let go both physically and mentally, that is to say, to eliminate the muscular and nervous tension which, after a certain time, produces what we call fatigue. Ten minutes of complete relaxation are equal to several hours of sleep. That is why all those who have an immense capacity for work withdraw by instinct for a few moments and rest when they are weary in body or mind.

The technique of relaxation is very simple. Lie on your back, legs straight, heels together, toes apart. The arms should fall naturally to the sides, a little away from them, and the hands with the palms upwards. The head should be held straight. Do not pick too soft a mattress. A blanket folded in two on the ground is just the thing. Undo your collar, loosen your belt, take off your shoes, remove your watch and glasses if you wear them. Nothing must impede the circulation of the blood nor press on any of the organs of the body. Then banish all extraneous thoughts and regulate your breathing with the first exercise already given. Next try, **while thinking about it intently**, to relax scalp, forehead, eyelids, nostrils, mouth, jaws, fingers completely and in that order. This is quite difficult at first but when you have succeeded all the rest of the body relaxes by itself without your having to think about it. Keep perfectly still. Act dead. Even in normal sleep the body remains tensed and the mind active. In this process of relaxation the mind must be in abeyance and the body must only function like a machine. The limbs must be supported only by the ground on which they rest, and its own weight must make the body sag completely (**Fig. 1**).

This is how complete relaxation is attained. You no longer think of anything. A sense of total well-being possesses you, and you are no longer aware of being yourself. And yet you are not asleep; you do not have to sleep. There you have complete rest, while your reserves of energy are used to make good the losses of the organism, while the relaxed brain lets the blood circulate more freely and eliminates the poisons produced by fatigue.

Practise the above for just a few minutes whenever you feel tired and, during the asana sessions, after each of them. During the latter, in fact, a great deal of energy is spent. The muscles and nerves are contracted. It is important, then, after each asana, to allow the organism time and opportunity to make up for what it has lost. The vital energy acquired by the practice of the asanas must be allowed to spread to the internal organs instead of going to be used up in the muscles.

SALUTE TO THE SUN

CHAPTER IV

Preliminary Exercise

THE movement which we are now going to describe is in a way a limbering-up exercise. It is essential to practise it at the beginning and end of each asana exercise. It is worth doing it, too, every morning when you awake. The blood is distributed to all the organs, the circulation is got going, and the state of sleepiness is banished. The nervous system is regulated, the eyes become brighter, the brain is cleared, and the whole appearance becomes as though glowing with health. This is the most complete physical exercise and we may say the most wonderful that there is, in the sense that it is a harmonious combination of breathing and the main asanas. It is a composite movement.

Done at the start of the day, it will keep your body and mind fit. Done at the start of the asanas, it will limber up your muscles and make it easier for you to carry out the asanas.

In itself this exercise is worth almost all the others put together, and beginners will find great benefit in practising it for five minutes at a time, at least twice a day for some weeks before starting the asanas proper.

Independently of the other asanas, this exercise, if practised daily, is enough to guarantee you a supple body and sound health. **It is the most important asana in Yoga.**

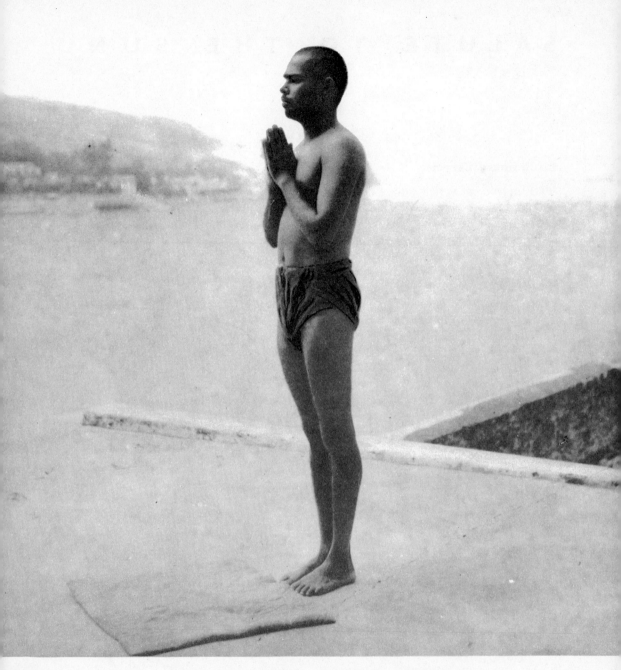

1. Stand up, hands together at chest level, feet together (**Fig. 2**).

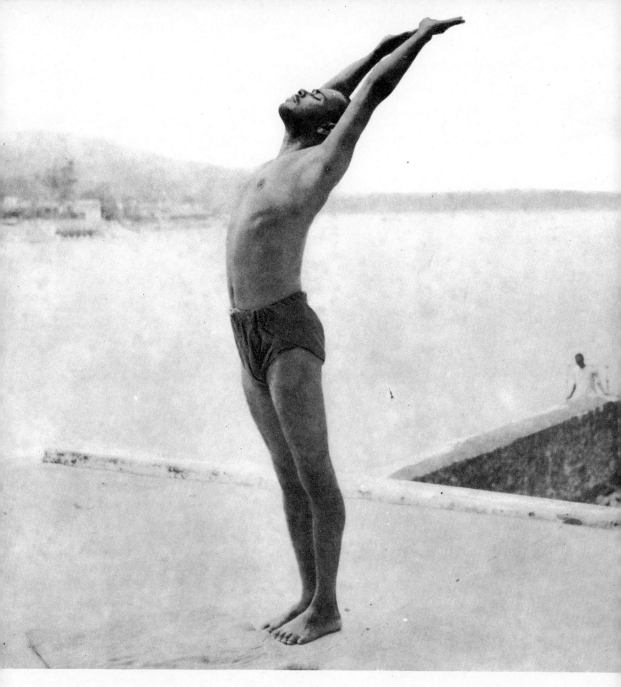

2. Raise the arms and the head as high as possible while **breathing in deeply (Fig. 3).**

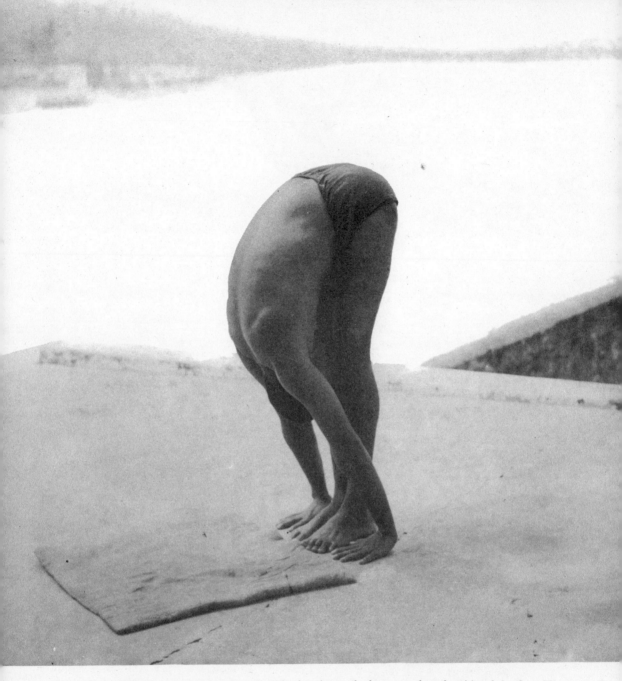

3. Bend the body forward so that the hands touch the ground at the side of the feet. The head should touch the knees, the legs remain straight. **Breathe out (Fig. 4).**

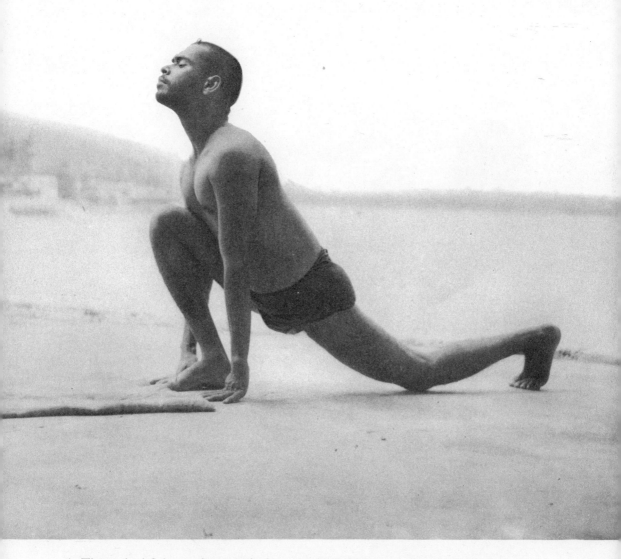

4. Throw the left leg to the rear, the knee touching the ground. Bend the right leg and press the foot on the ground. Raise the chin as high as possible. **Keep the lungs empty (Fig. 5).**

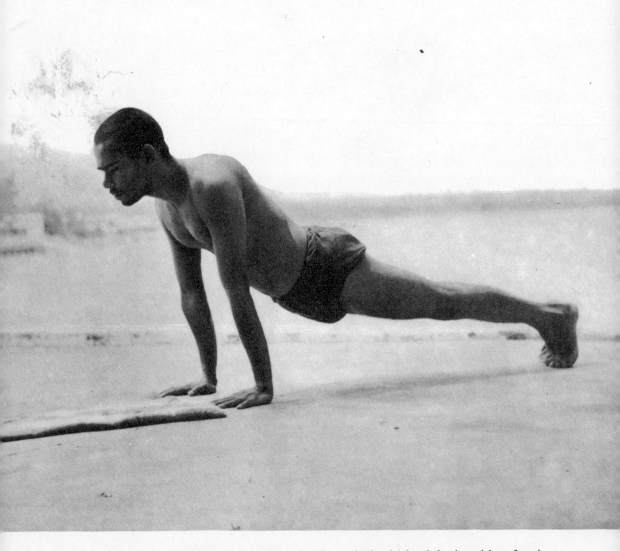

5. Throw the right leg back as well, and make a plank; the head, back and legs forming a straight line, the arms extended. **Breathe in** (Fig. 6).

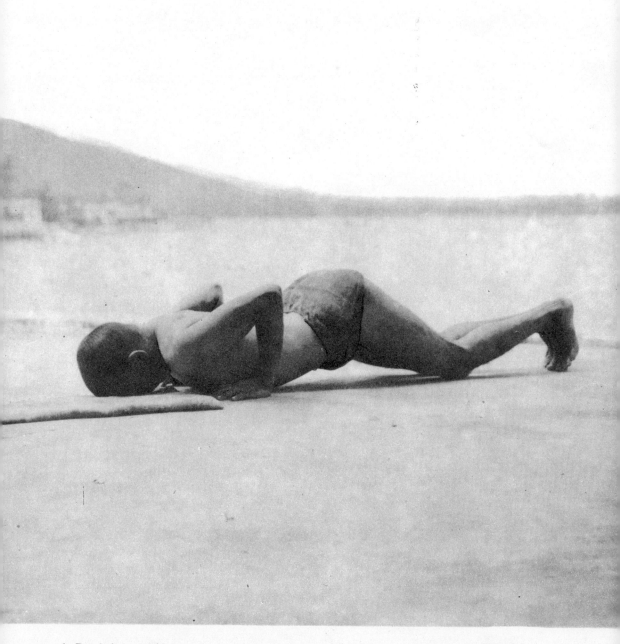

6. Bend the arms and let the body rest on the ground; only the forehead, chest, hands, knees and toes in contact with the ground. **Hold the breath (Fig. 7).**

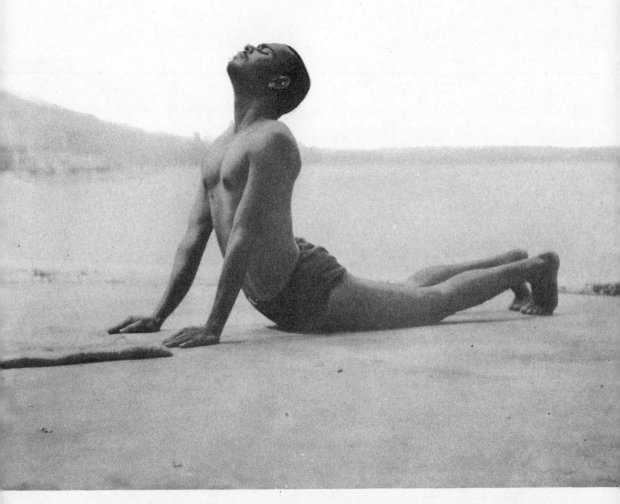

7. Raise the head and push on the arms so as to bring the trunk upright, the legs and pelvis staying on the ground. **Breathe out** (Fig. 8).

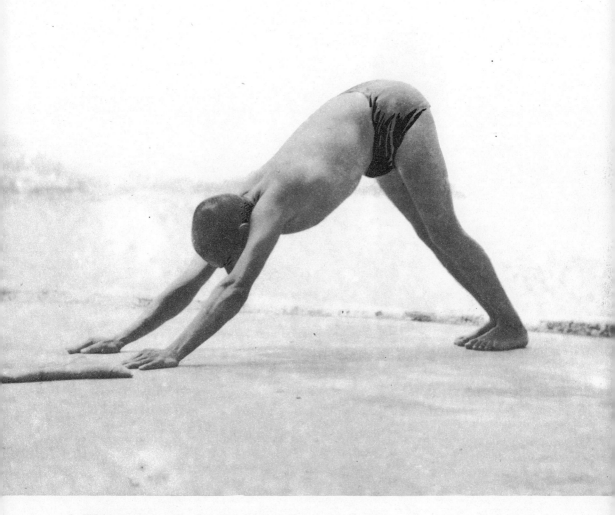

8. Without moving the feet and hands, raise the entire body again, arching the back. **Breathe in (Fig. 9).**

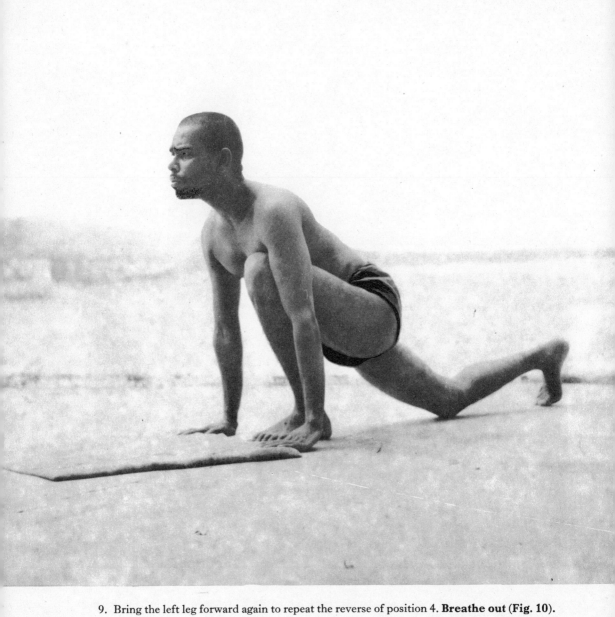

9. Bring the left leg forward again to repeat the reverse of position 4. **Breathe out (Fig. 10).**

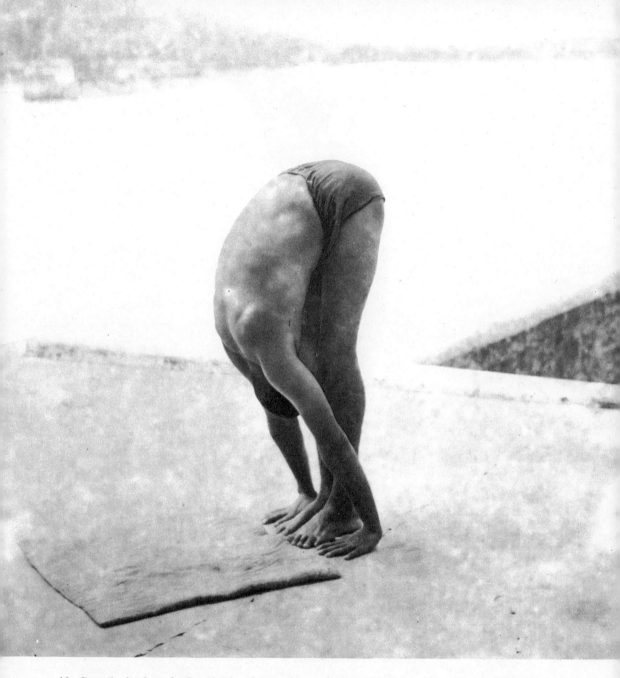

10. Stretch the legs, letting the hands remain on the ground to repeat position 3. **Keep the lungs empty (Fig. 11)**.

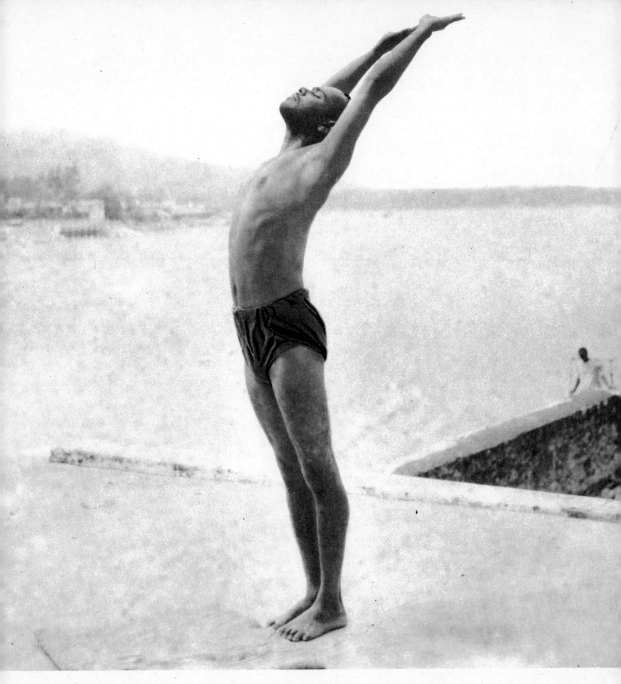

11. Return to position 2 and **breathe in** (Fig. 12).

ASANAS OF THE FIRST DEGREE

CHAPTER V

GROUP 1

Head Stand *(Sirshasana)*

TECHNIQUE

1. Kneel, put the forearms on the ground and clasp the hands with fingers interlocked. **Breathe out.**

2. Cushion the top of your head against your hands.

3. With a very light stretch of the legs raise your body, the toes staying on the ground.

4. Slowly raise the legs with them bent. **Breathe in.**

5. Stretch the legs up straight. **Breathe normally (Figs. 13, 14, 15).**

This is not very difficult to achieve. After a few attempts you will succeed very well with this movement. If you are afraid of falling backwards, get someone to help you or else support yourself against a wall. When you have learned to keep your balance and can stay like that for some seconds, try to keep completely still. Start with five seconds, then ten, and increase regularly, yet without remaining long enough for the blood to run to the head. After that come back very slowly to your first position and stand still for ten seconds. Then take a rest. This advice applies to all the asanas.

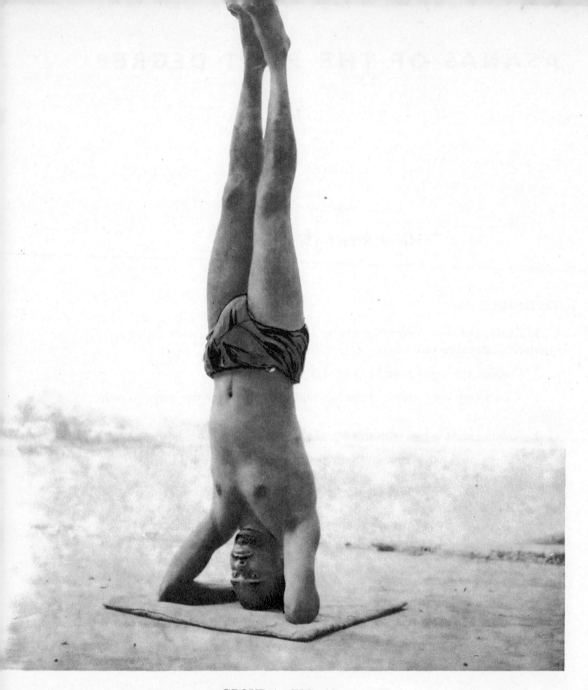

GROUP 1 – FIG. 13
Head Stand *(Sirshasana)*

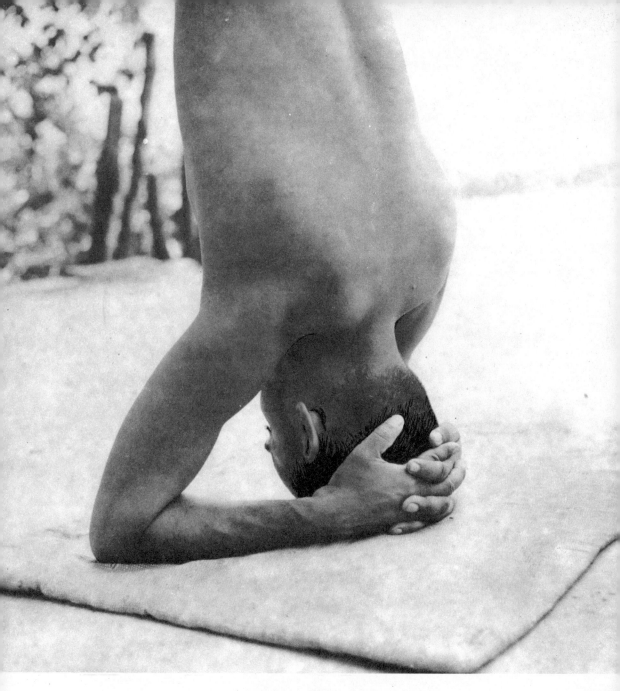

GROUP 1 – FIG. 14
Head Stand
Detail showing the position of the hands.

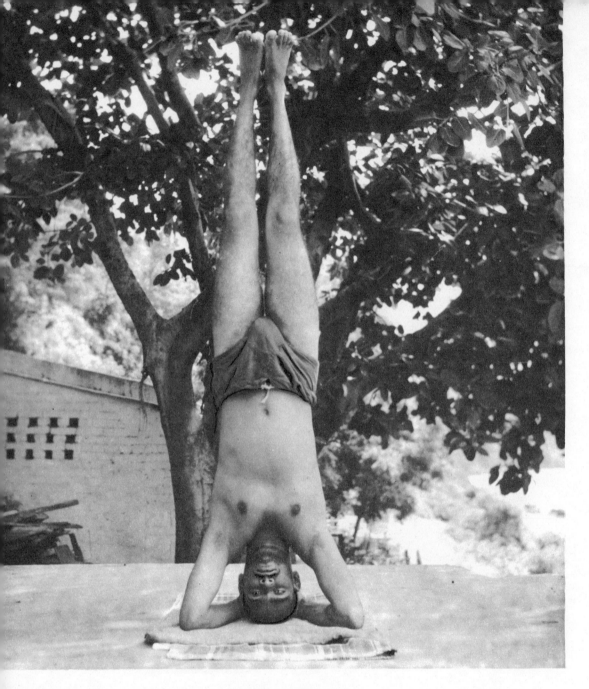

GROUP 1 – FIG. 15
Head Stand
Front

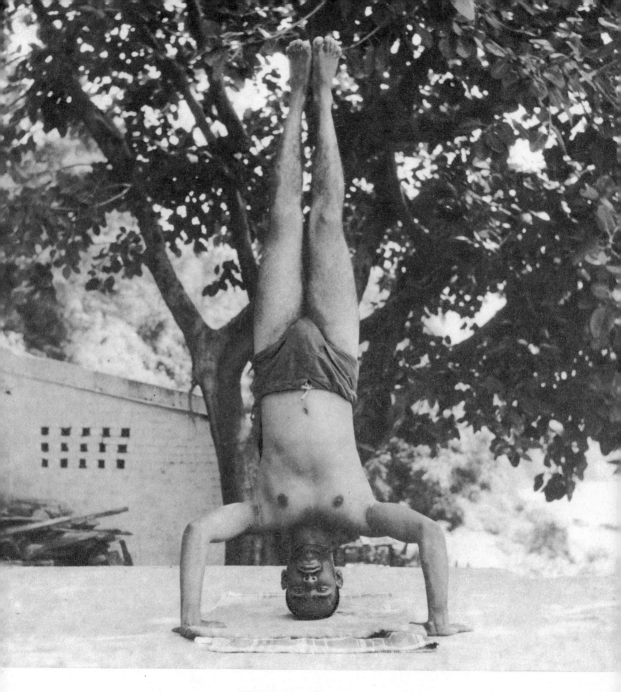

GROUP 1 – FIG. 16
Tree Asana

Instead of resting the forearms on the ground, you can also put just the hands. This is **Vrikshasana, the tree posture (Fig. 16).**

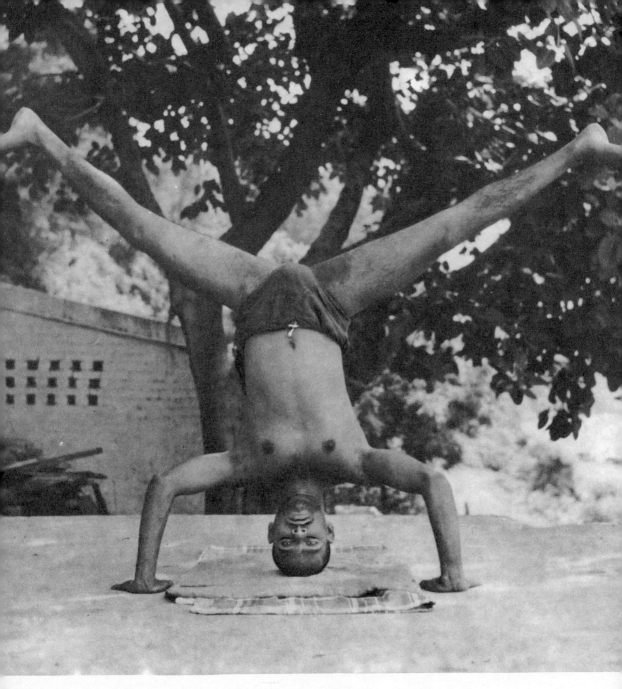

GROUP 1 – FIG. 17
Tree Asana
Variation
In this position you can spread the legs slowly, then bring them together again (**Fig. 17**).

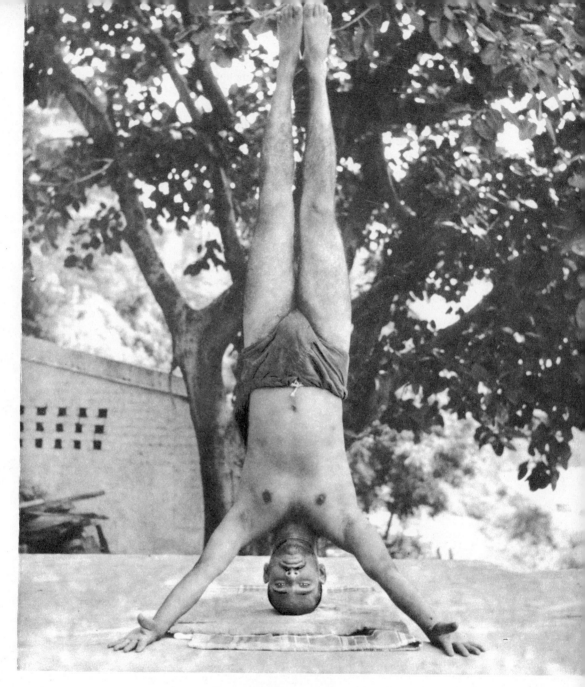

GROUP 1 – FIG. 18

Tree Asana

Variation

Or else—and this is more difficult—you can stretch out the arms and rest only on the head and the back of the hands. This develops your sense of balance (**Fig. 18**).

RESULTS

The aorta, the carotids and the subclavian arteries receive an increase of arterial blood. The brain, the spinal cord and the sympathetic nervous system are supplied with a constant flow. Disorders of the nerves, eyes, ears, nose and throat disappear rapidly. This asana is a marvellous remedy for varicose veins, renal colic and stubborn constipation. Memory and brain capacity are increased. Neurasthenia disappears. This asana is excellent for combating dropped stomach, rupture in the early stages, and nervous or hepatic asthma.

CONTRA-INDICATIONS

This asana should not be used in cases of head noises, facial neuralgia, sanguine temperaments with naturally bloodshot eyes, and chronic nasal catarrh. **Never** practise this asana immediately after strenuous exercise. Wait for half an hour.

Complete Asana *(Sarvangasana)*

TECHNIQUE

1. Lie on your back.

2. Slowly raise the legs straight up.

3. Put your hands on the hips and with the aid of the latter raise the body vertically.

4. Keep the body raised in this position. The chin should touch the chest, the elbows rest on the ground. **Breathe through the nose** and from the stomach.

5. Take a rest **(Fig. 19)**.

Try to perform the variations of a single movement one after the other slowly then return to the main position and rest.

RESULTS

This asana strengthens the thyroid gland and in that way the whole body, too, the thyroid being the most important endocrine gland. This posture helps the user to keep a youthful figure and a smooth skin, and women will find great benefit in it. Seminal losses, indigestion, constipation, varicose veins and stomach troubles disappear. The spine is kept flexible and premature stiffness warded off.

CONTRA-INDICATIONS

These are the same as for the head stand.

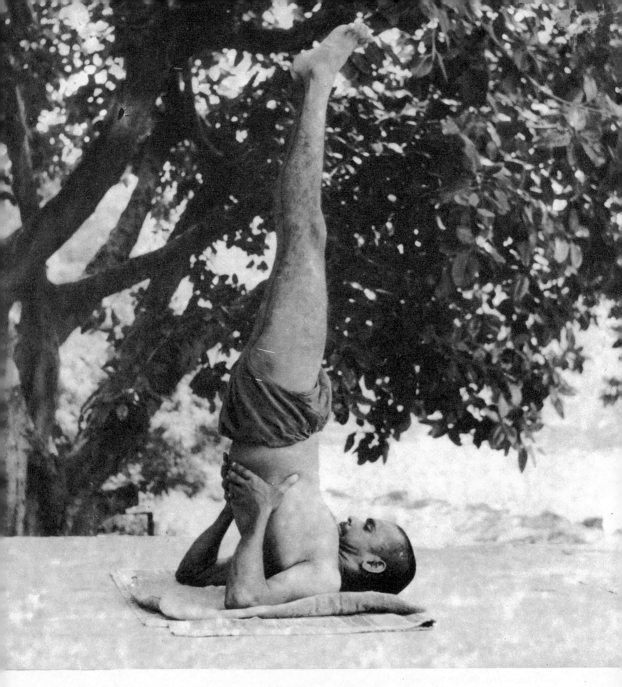

GROUP 2 – FIG. 19
Sarvangasana or **Complete Asana**

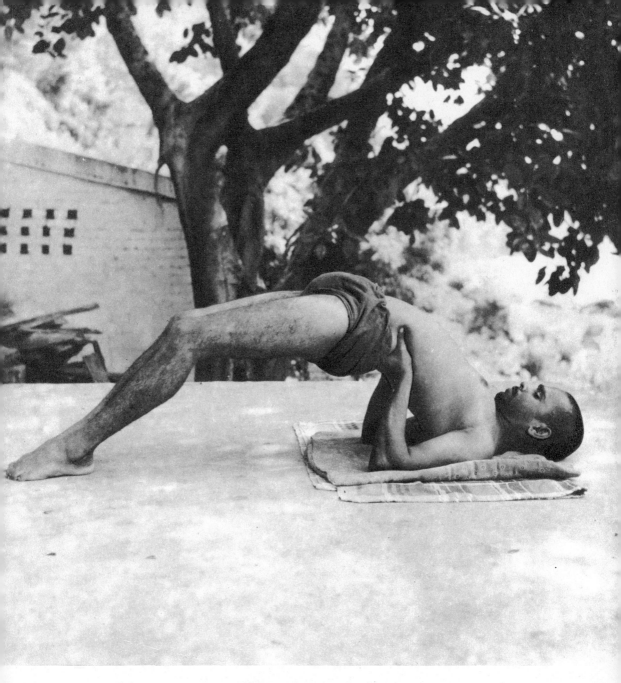

GROUP 2 – FIG. 20

Sarvangasana

Variations

(A) **Sedhubandhasana.** In the Complete Asana position (**Fig. 19**) bring the legs down slowly until the feet touch the ground. This is the **Bridge Asana (Fig. 20)**.

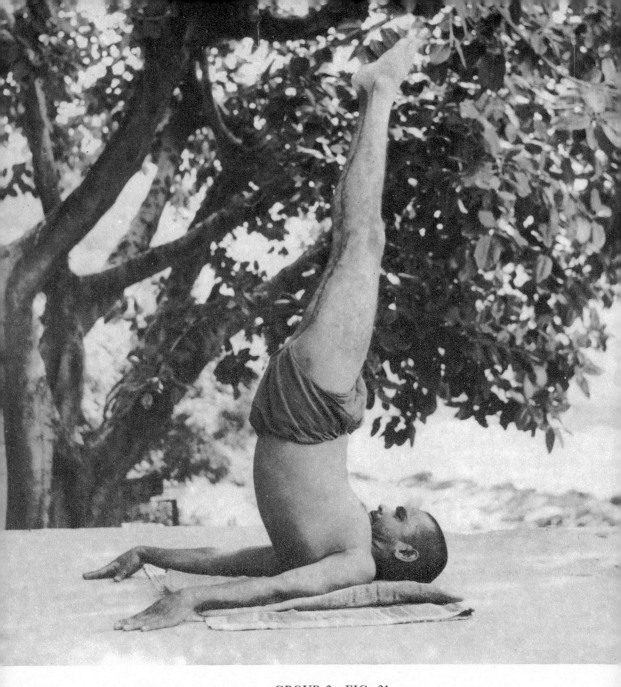

GROUP 2 – FIG. 21

(B) **Variation of Sarvangasana.** In the Complete Asana position (**Fig. 19**) release the hands and spread them on the ground (**Fig. 21**).

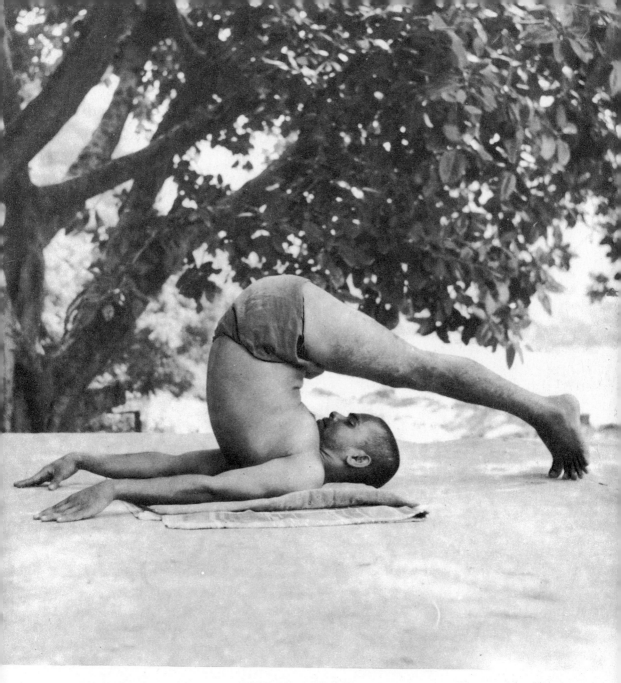

GROUP 2 – FIG. 22

(C) **Variation of Sarvangasana. Halasana (1).** In the previous position (**Fig. 21**) touch the ground behind your head with the toes, stretching as far as possible. This is the **Plough Asana (Fig. 22).**

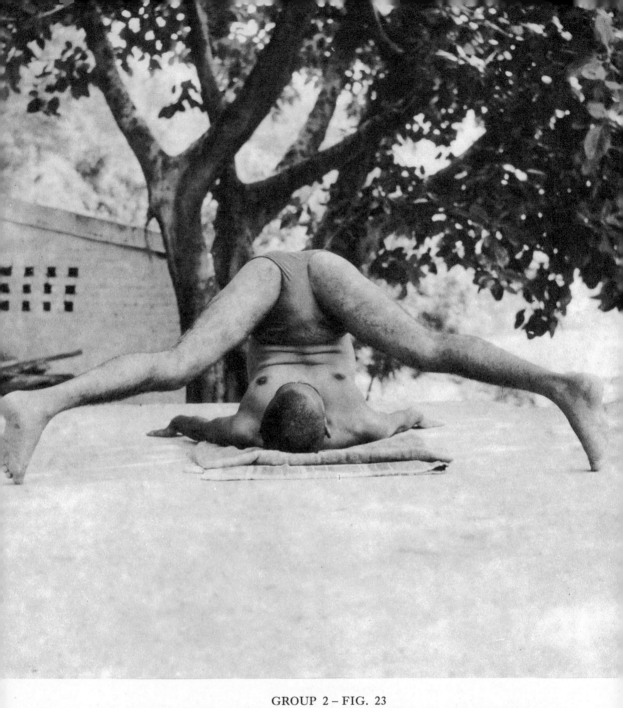

GROUP 2 – FIG. 23

(D) **Variation of Halasana (2).** Same as **Fig. 22,** but with the legs spread apart (**Fig. 23**).

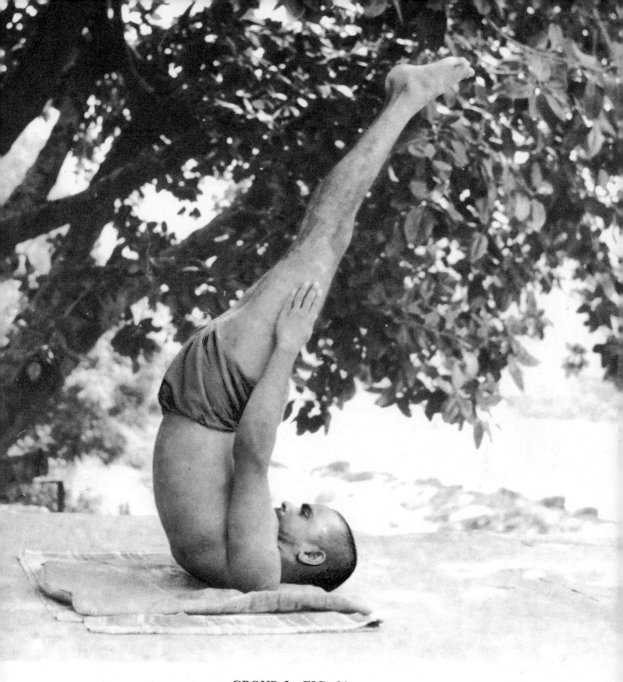

GROUP 2 – FIG. 24

(E) **Variation of Sarvangasana.** In the first position (**Fig. 19**) release the hands and lay them by the sides. Retain the balance (**Fig. 24**).

GROUP 3

Wheel Asana (*Chakrasana*)

TECHNIQUE

1. Lie on the back.

2. Bend the legs and place the hands flat on the ground behind the shoulders (**Fig. 25**).

3. Lift your body as high as possible **while taking deep breaths** (**Fig. 26**).

4. Keep this position for a few seconds **while holding your breath**.

5. Resume the starting position **as you breathe out**.

We commonly call this asana **"the Bridge."** Repeat it three or four times running.

VARIANTS

Kneeling on the ground, lean back and rest your extended arms on your ankles. This is the **Asana of Firmness (Dhrityasana)** (**Fig. 27**).

Repeat this variant while standing up. Bend the head back as far as possible (**Fig. 28**).

RESULTS

These asanas strengthen the muscles of the abdomen, thighs and legs. They make the loins supple, improve the memory, and cure affections of the trachea and larynx.

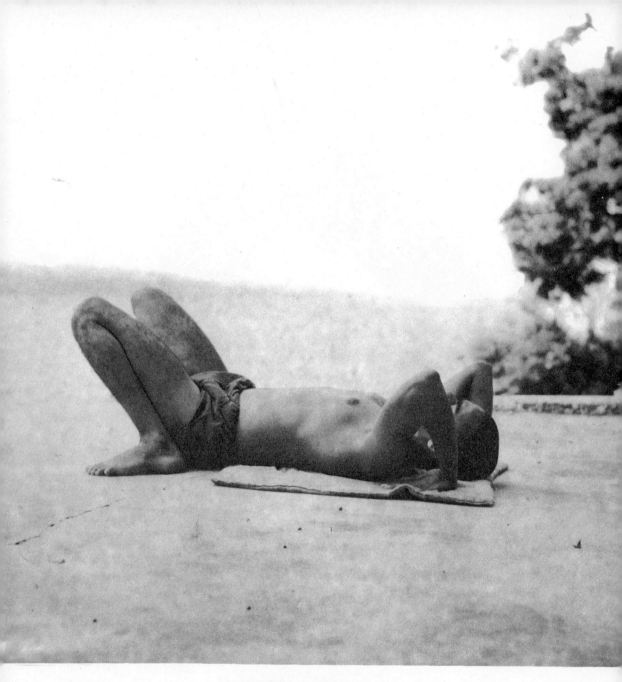

GROUP 3 – FIG. 25
Wheel Asana *(Chakrasana)*
Starting position.

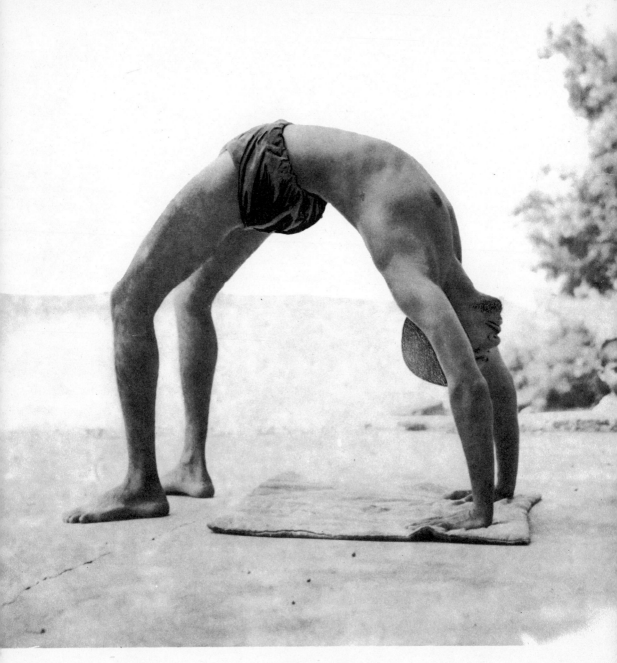

GROUP 3 – FIG. 26
Wheel Asana

54

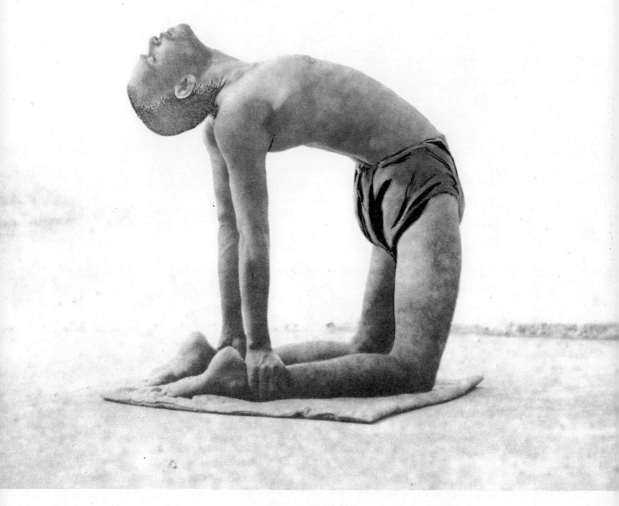

GROUP 3 – FIG. 27

First variation of the **Wheel Asana,** known as: Asana of Firmness *(Dhrityasana)*

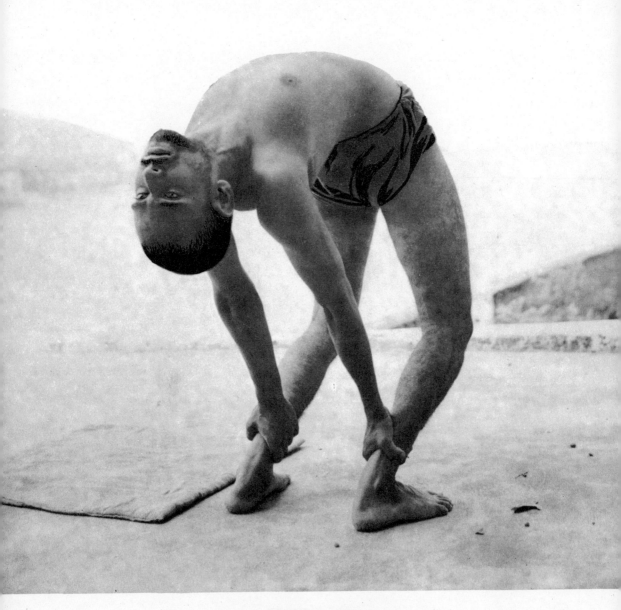

GROUP 3 – FIG. 28.
Second variation of the **Wheel Asana**.

Bow Asana *(Dhanurasana)*

TECHNIQUE

1. Lie flat on your stomach with the arms by the sides.

2. Bend the legs, bringing the heels to the thighs.

3. Grasp your ankles with the hands (**Fig. 29**).

4. **As you breathe in** stretch legs and arms so as to arch your body, which should rest only on the abdomen. Keep the knees together. **Hold** the position and **the breath** for a few seconds (**Fig. 30**).

5. Return slowly to the first position **as you breathe out**. Start this asana again three or four times running.

RESULTS

This asana gives the same results as the two preceding ones. It is specially recommended for women. It rids them of surplus fat round the buttocks and stomach and on the hips and thighs. It gives a firm bust and develops shapely breasts. It strengthens the trapezoid muscles.

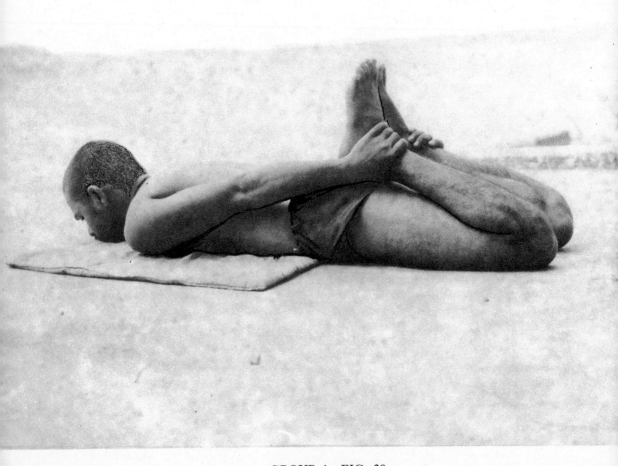

GROUP 4 – FIG. 29
Bow Asana
Starting position.

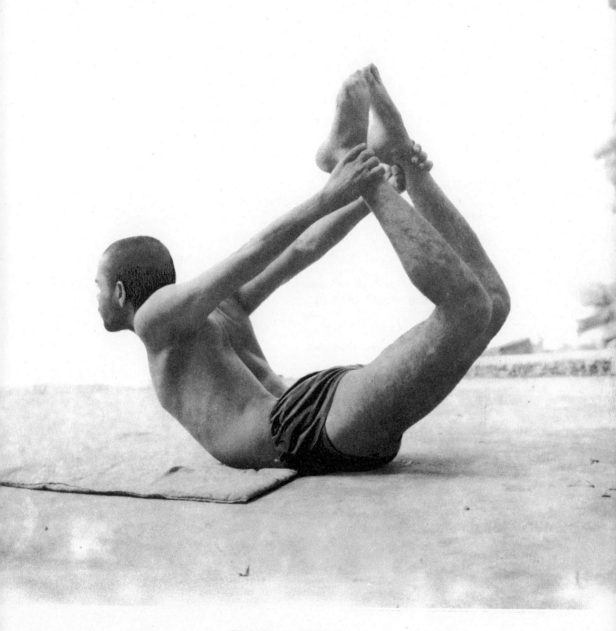

GROUP 4 – FIG. 30
Bow Asana

59

Cobra Asana *(Bhujangasana)*

TECHNIQUE

1. Lie flat on your stomach.

2. Place your hands flat under your shoulders.

3. Raise the body slowly until the arms are extended, **while you breathe in**.

4. Hold the head as high as possible. The thighs should touch the ground all the time. **Hold the breath (Fig. 31)**.

5. Come back very gently to the crouching position, **breathing out**.

Repeat five or six times, then rest.

RESULTS

The muscles of the back are massaged and strengthened, also those of the abdomen. The abdominal pressure thus created combats constipation.

This asana also combats amenorrhoea, dysmenorrhoea, leucorrhoea and other women's complaints.

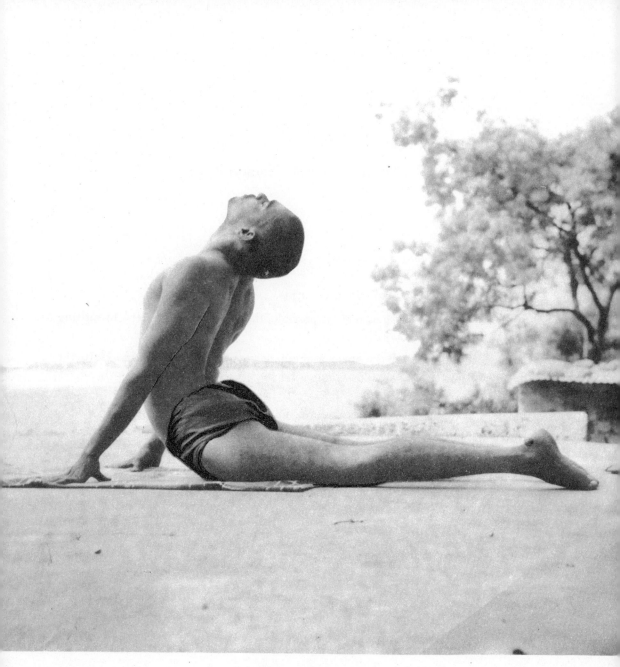

GROUP 5 – FIG. 31
Cobra Asana

GROUP 6

Locust Asana *(Salabhasana)*

TECHNIQUE

1. Lie on the stomach, arms by the sides, palms uppermost.

2. Clench the fists and stiffen the arms.

3. Raise the right leg as high as possible, then the left, alternately, **breathing rhythmically** (**Fig. 32**).

4. Legs together. Raise them as high as possible, **breathing in**. **Hold** the position and **the breath** for a few seconds, then lower yourself slowly to the ground, **breathing out** (**Fig. 33**).

Repeat that five or six times running. Rest.

RESULTS

As in the preceding asana, the abdominal pressure is greatly increased, and this regulates the intestinal functions and strengthens the resistance of the abdominal walls. The liver, pancreas and kidneys are massaged. Back pains and sciatica are banished in a short time.

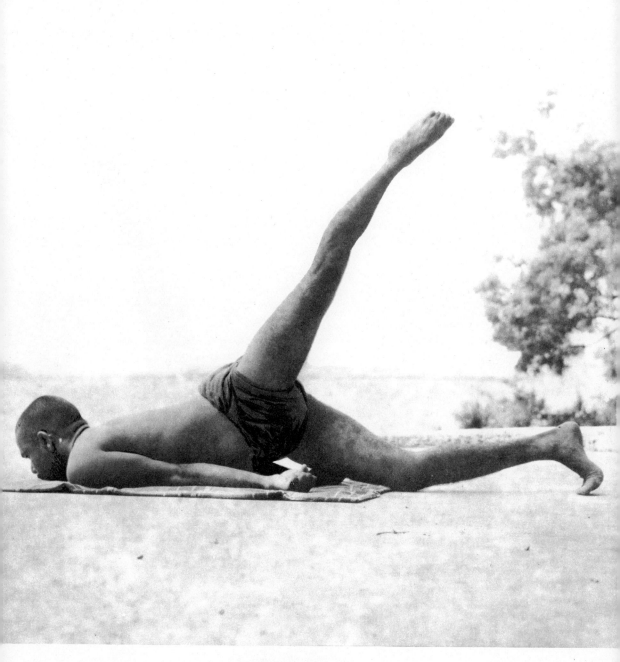

GROUP 6 – FIG. 32
Locust Asana
(Semi-position)

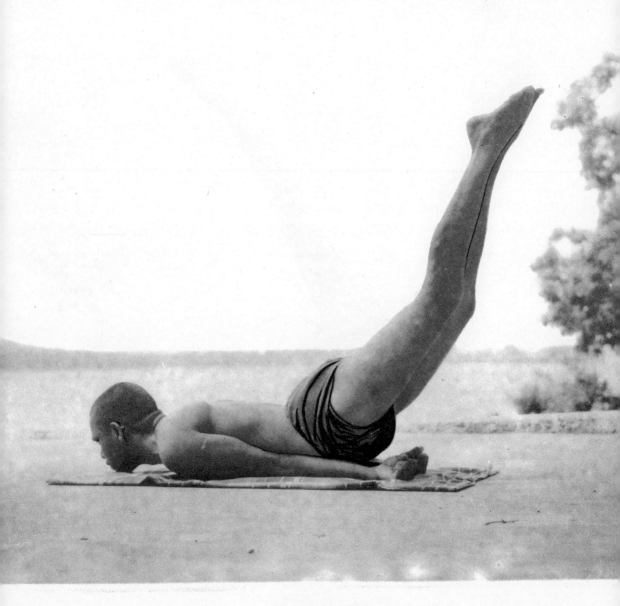

GROUP 6 – FIG. 33
Locust Asana
(Full position)

GROUP 7

Triangle Asana *(Trikonasana)*

TECHNIQUE

1. Stand up, legs apart, arms stretched out at shoulder height. **Breathe in.**

2. Bend your body to the side so as to touch the toes with the hand, arms and legs extended. **Breathe out (Fig. 34).**

3. Come back to the first position, **breathing in** again. Do the same movement alternately to right and left.

VARIATIONS

Do the same movement, but with turning of the trunk to touch the feet with the opposite hand (**Fig. 35**), or bending one leg (**Figs. 36, 37**).

RESULTS

Better working of the bowels. Gives an appetite and assists digestion. The muscles of the trunk and back are made supple. Attacks of backache are avoided, the liver is massaged and secretes more abundantly.

E

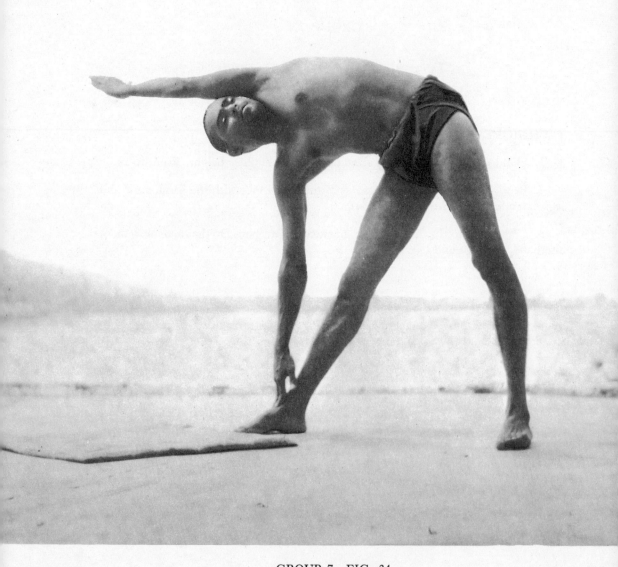

GROUP 7 – FIG. 34
Triangle Asana
Basic

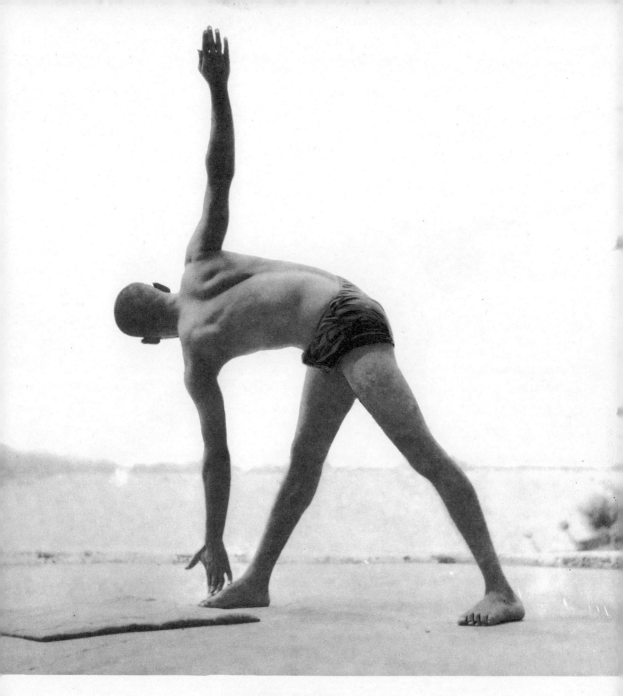

GROUP 7 – FIG. 35
Triangle Asana
Turn to right

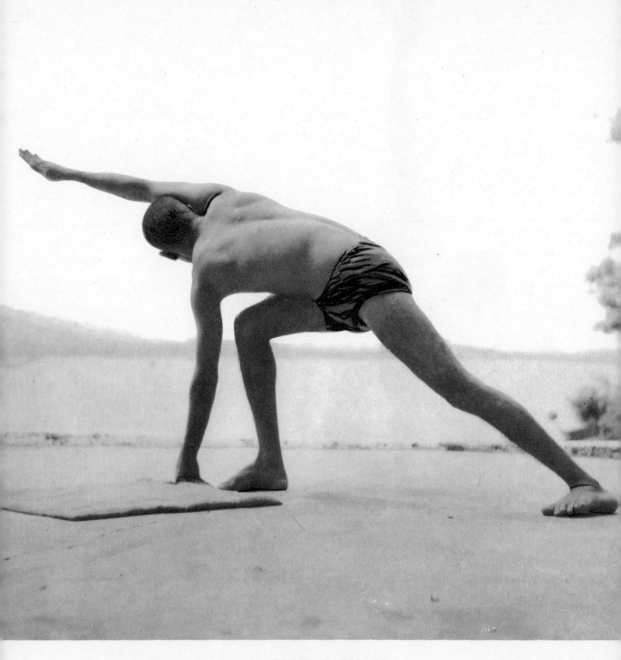

GROUP 7 – FIG. 36
Triangle Asana
Bending to right

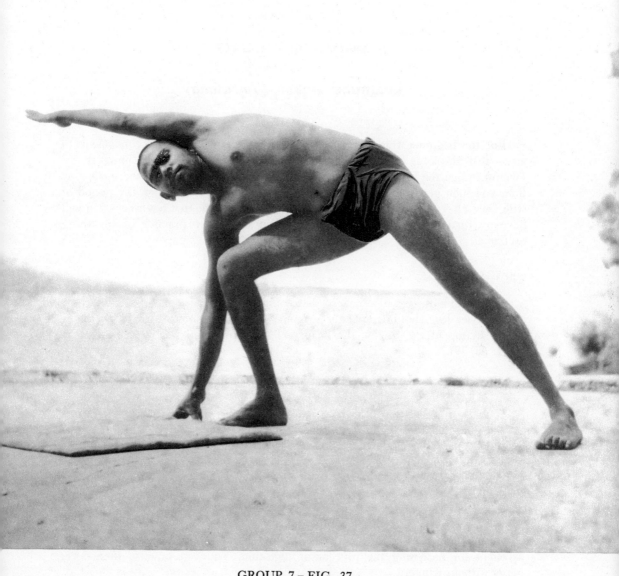

GROUP 7 – FIG. 37
Triangle Asana
Simple Bending

GROUP 8

ASANAS OF STABILITY

Diamond Asana (Vajrasana)

For the beginner this position will be more comfortable and convenient to attain than the lotus or Buddha pose. It will prepare for the latter, however, by making supple the synovial ligaments (knee-joint) and the joint of the instep. At first, you soon get tired and stiff. Don't try too hard, but lengthen the period of stillness each day, even if only for a few seconds at a time. In a few weeks you will have no further trouble. This position is ideal for the practice of breathing exercises.

TECHNIQUE

Just kneel with legs together, so that you are sitting on your heels. The whole of the lower legs should touch the ground. The hands should rest flat, without effort, on top of the thighs, the head and trunk remaining in a vertical plane (**Figs. 38, 39**).

VARIATIONS

While in this position, lean back, supporting yourself with the arms, and rest the back and head on the ground. The knees must not be raised. Cross the arms behind the head like a pillow or else leave them at the sides (**Figs. 40, 41**).

You can also sit in the diamond posture, but opening the knees as wide apart as possible. This is then the **Frog Asana (Mandukasana)** (**Fig. 42**).

RESULTS

By reducing the flow of blood into the lower limbs, these simple postures are excellent for hastening the process of digestion. You can practise them after meals without danger.

These asanas of stability and stillness assist breath-control and mental concentration. That is why orientals use them so often.

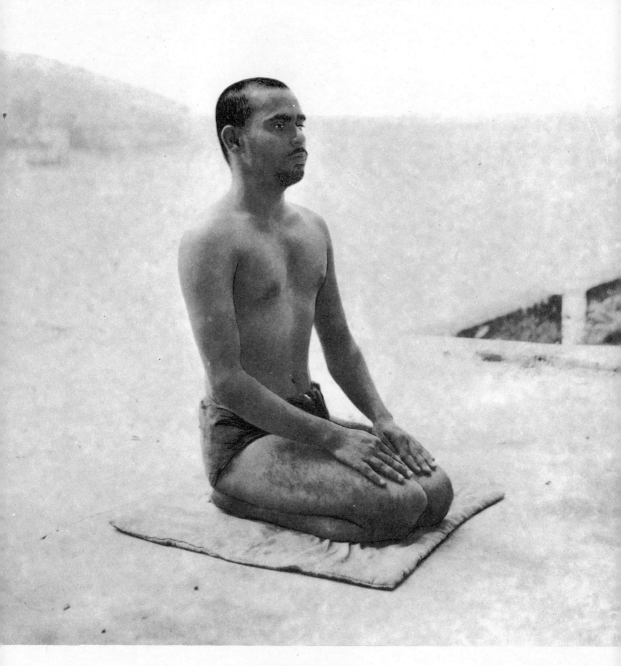

GROUP 8 – FIG. 38
Diamond Asana
Front

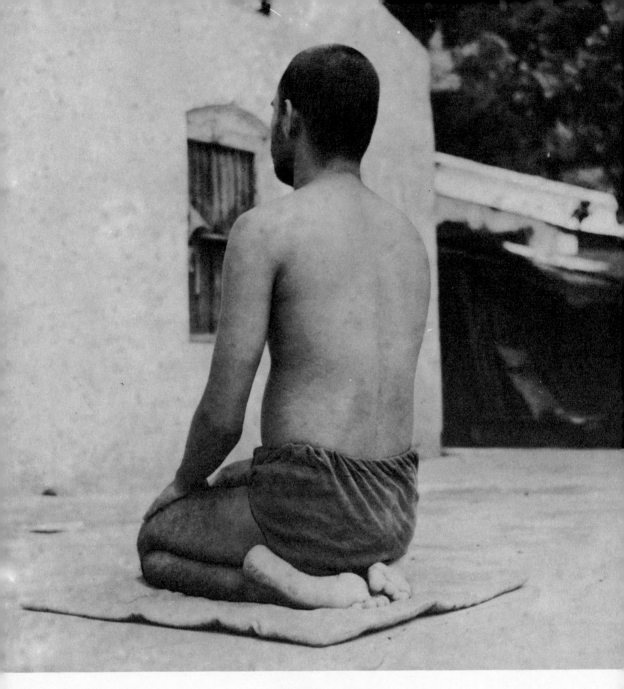

GROUP 8 – FIG. 39
Diamond Asana
Rear

72

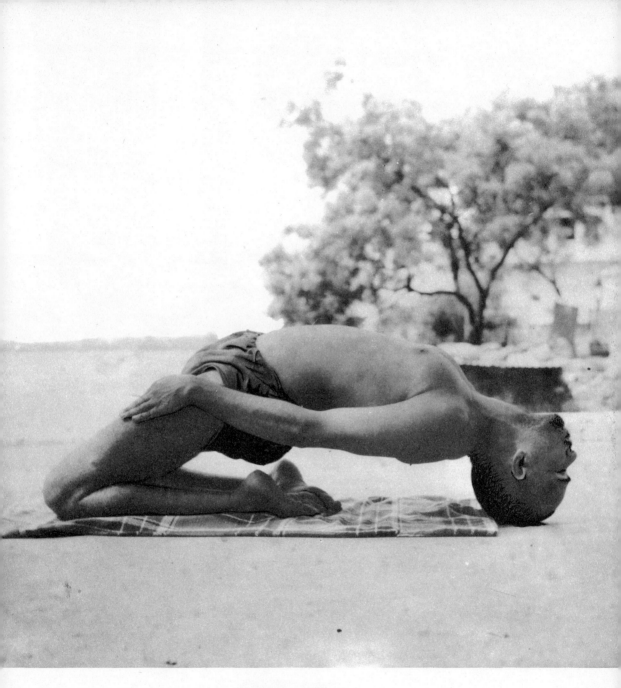

GROUP 8 – FIG. 40
Diamond Asana
Supine. First position

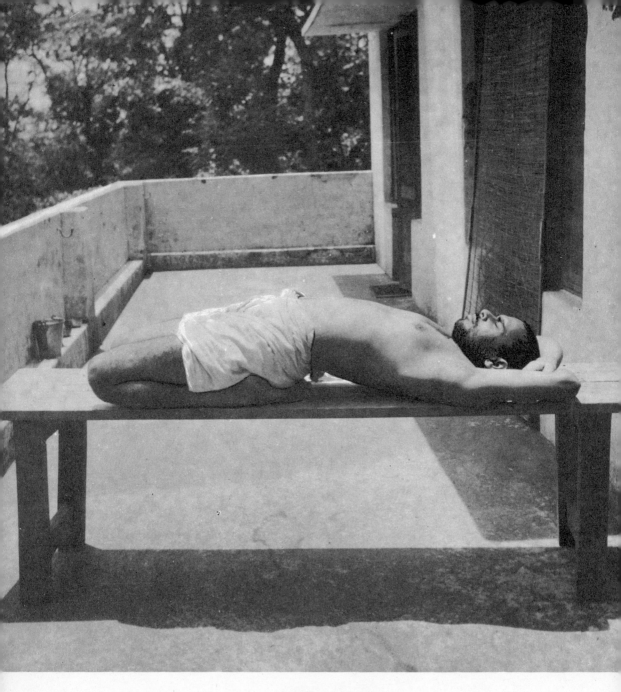

GROUP 8 – FIG. 41
Diamond Asana
Supine. Second position

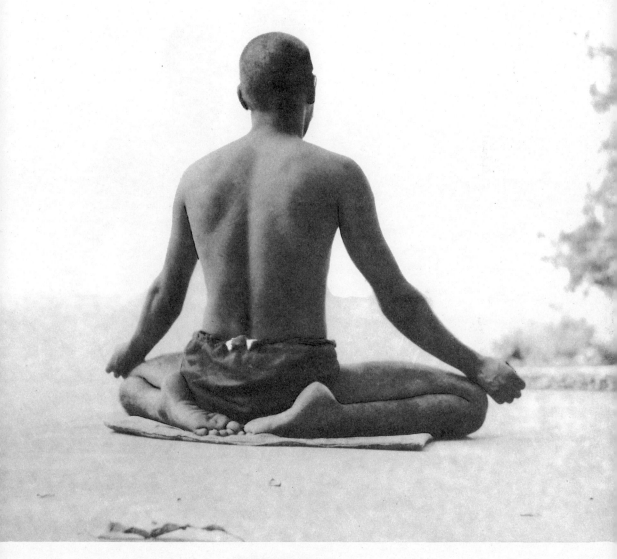

GROUP 8 – FIG. 42
Frog Asana

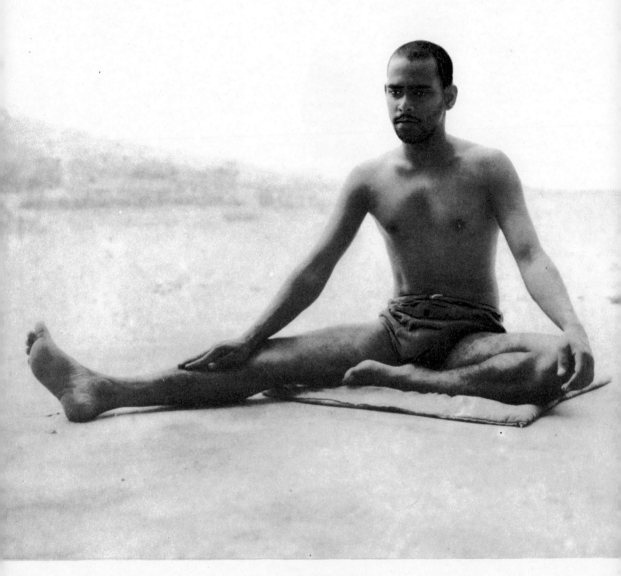

GROUP 8 – FIG. 43
Disciple Asana

Finally, we prescribe for you another pose, which is very easy for the beginner to adopt: sit down, body straight, legs apart, then bring back one of your legs and wedge the foot against the inside of the other calf. This is **"Sidhasana,"** the **disciple posture**.

76

GROUP 9

Pincers Asana *(Paschimottanasana)*

TECHNIQUE

1. Lie on the back, arms extended by the sides. **Breathe in.**

2. Bend the whole body and grasp the big toes with your hands **as you breathe out (Fig. 44).**

3. Pull on the arms and touch your knees with your forehead. **Keep your lungs empty.**

4. Return slowly to the starting position **while breathing in.**

Repeat that several times in succession.

VARIATIONS

You can repeat the same exercise while standing up (**Figs. 45, 46**).

It is easier still to stand with legs apart and, with arms crossed behind the back, try to touch one of your knees with the forehead. This is then **Konasana**, the **angle posture (Fig. 47).**

RESULTS

These exercises stretch the body and all the muscles, make the spinal column supple and take fat off the stomach. The lymphatic system is made young and strong again. The stomach muscles are strengthened. Sciatica can be avoided.

Never keep this position longer than three minutes.

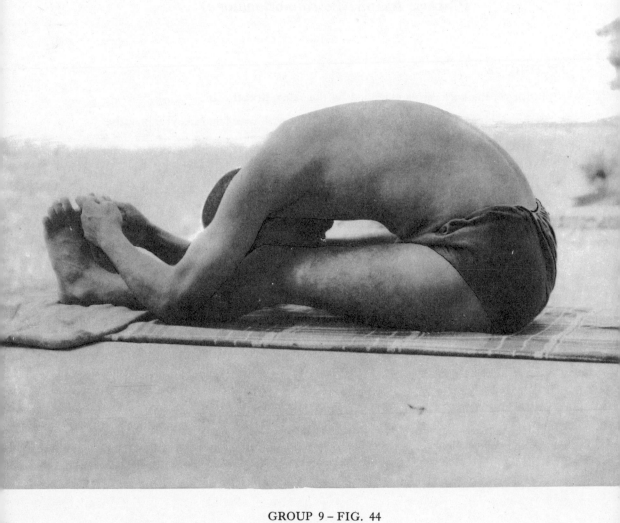

GROUP 9 – FIG. 44
Pincers Asana
Sitting

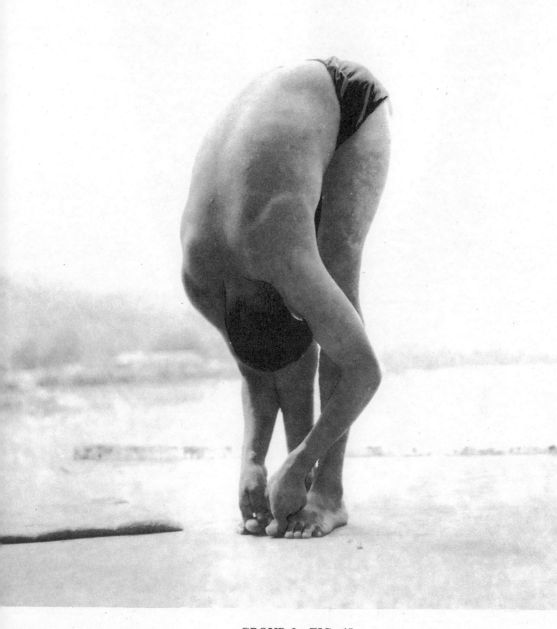

GROUP 9 – FIG. 45
Pincers Asana
Standing

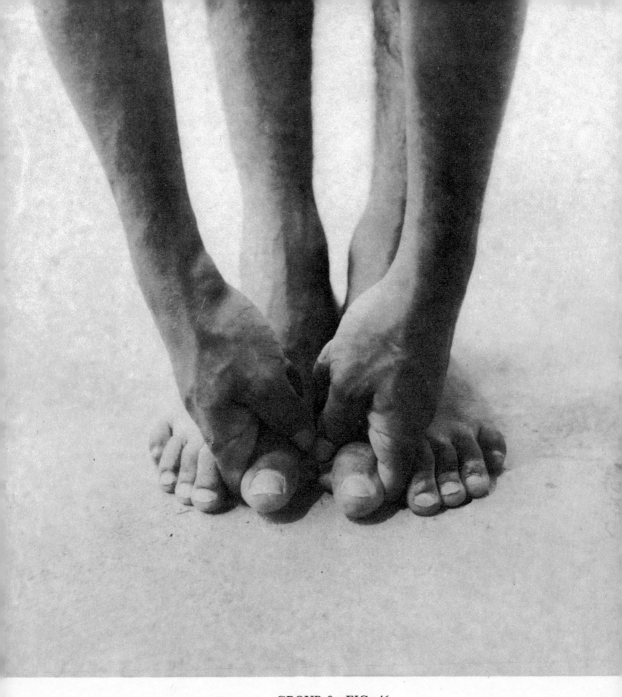

GROUP 9 – FIG. 46
Pincers Asana
Detail of the hands

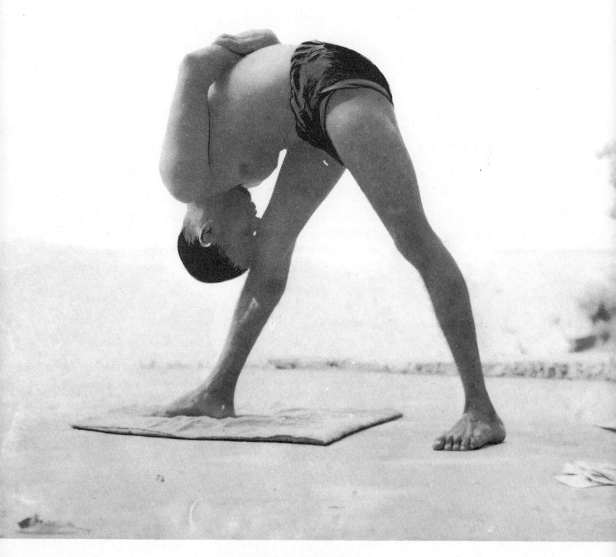

GROUP 9 – FIG. 47
Angle Asana *(Konasana)*

GROUP 10

Raven Asana *(Kakasana)*

TECHNIQUE

1. Lean forward and place both hands on the ground, about 18 inches apart.

2. Put the inside of the legs near the knee on the muscles at the back of the arms. The feet should touch together at the toes.

3. Try to keep your balance as you raise the feet and lean forward. **Breathe gently**, then return to your starting position (**Fig. 48**).

VARIANTS

Try to perform the same movement with both legs together and resting the thighs on one arm (**Figs. 49, 50**).

Or else you can find your balance, too, while resting the inside of the thighs on one arm and crossing the feet scissorswise. This is the **Asana of the Eight Curves** or **Astha Vakrasana (Fig. 51**).

RESULTS

These asanas strengthen the muscles of the hands, arms and shoulders. They assist mental concentration and blood circulation in the neck and face.

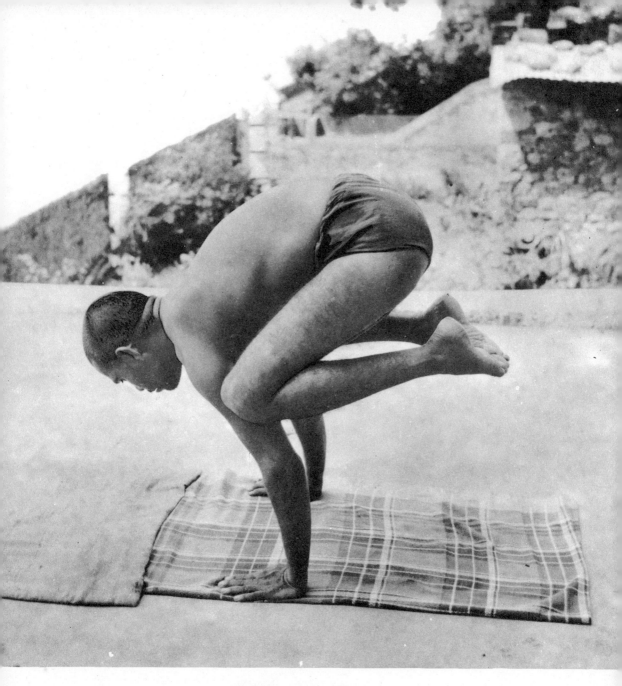

GROUP 10 – FIG. 48
Raven Asana

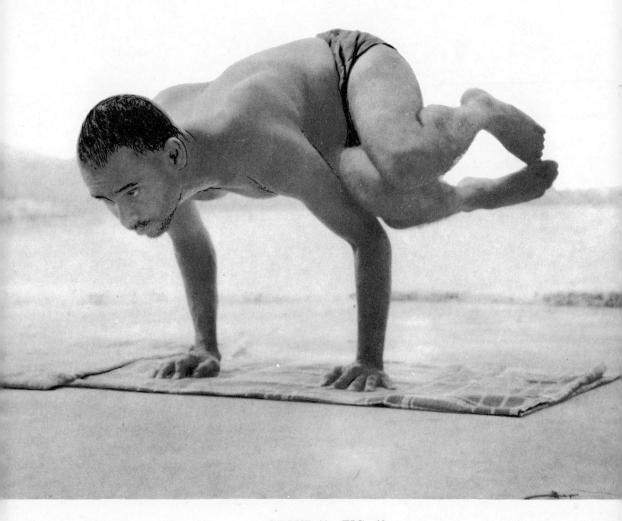

GROUP 10 – FIG. 49
Raven Asana
Left variation

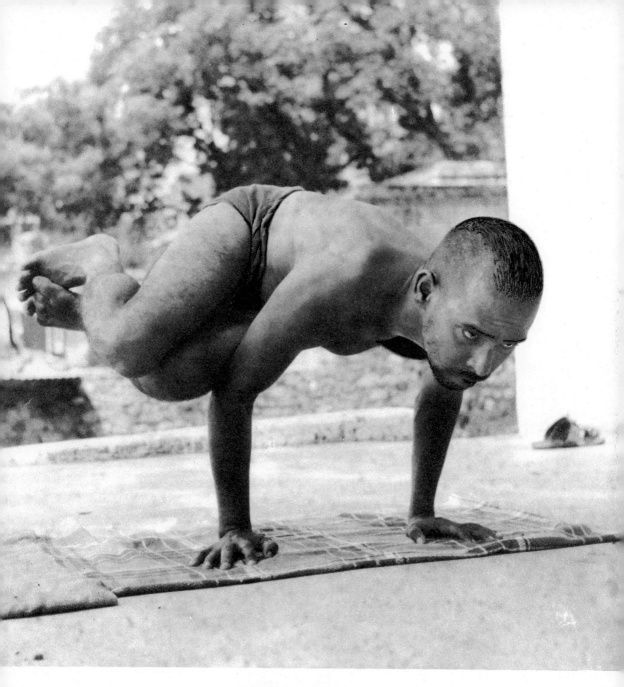

GROUP 10 – FIG. 50
Raven Asana
Right variation

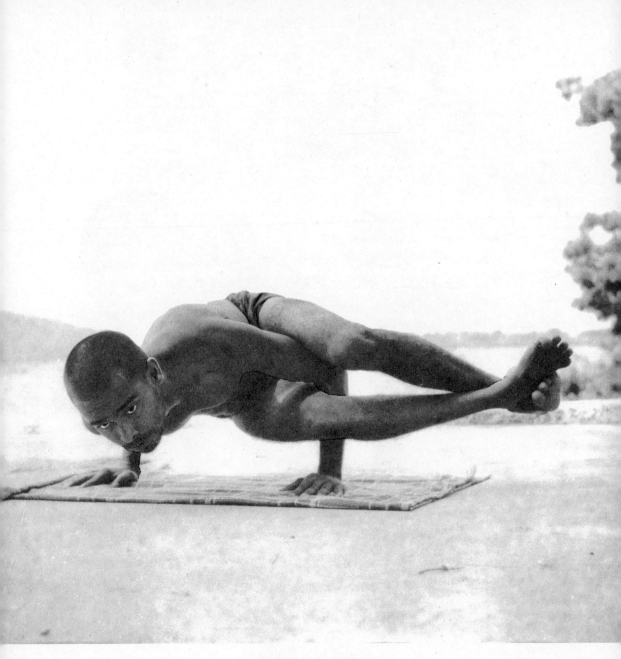

GROUP 10 – FIG. 51
Asana of the Eight Curves

GROUP 11

Peacock Asana *(Mayurasana)*

TECHNIQUE

1. Kneel on the ground.

2. Place the flat of the hands between the knees, with the fingers pointing towards the body and keeping the elbows together (**Fig. 52**).

3. Lean forward and stretch the legs out.

4. Lean farther forward and try to lift the legs from the ground, balancing the body and **taking a deep breath**. The elbows should press into the stomach. **Breathe gently** and keep the posture as long as possible (**Fig. 53**).

VARIATIONS

To strengthen the muscles of the hands, wrists and forearms, you can support yourself on your open hands with thumbs reversed, or even on the closed fists, but this is very difficult (**Figs. 54, 55**).

RESULTS

The abdominal aorta being partially compressed by the elbows, the flow of blood assists the digestive organs, toning up the liver, stomach and pancreas. This exercise acts rapidly to restore the nervous system.

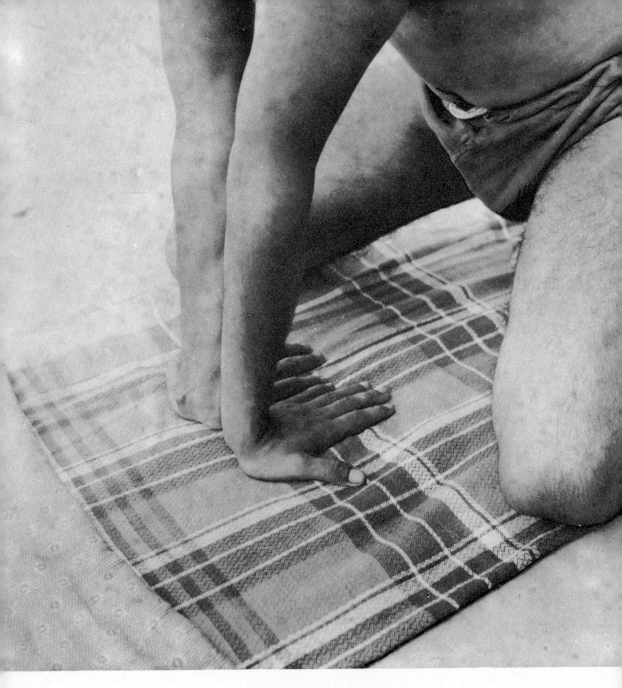

GROUP 11 – FIG. 52
Peacock Asana
Normal position of hands

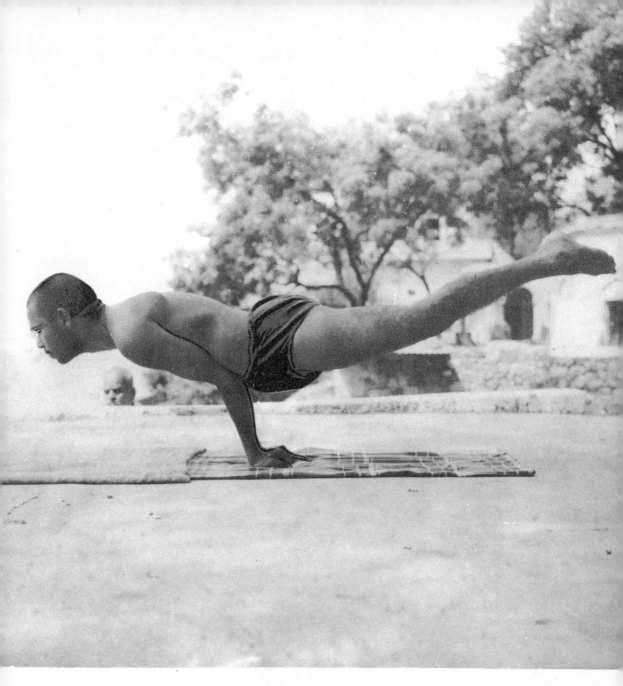

GROUP 11 – FIG. 53
Peacock Asana

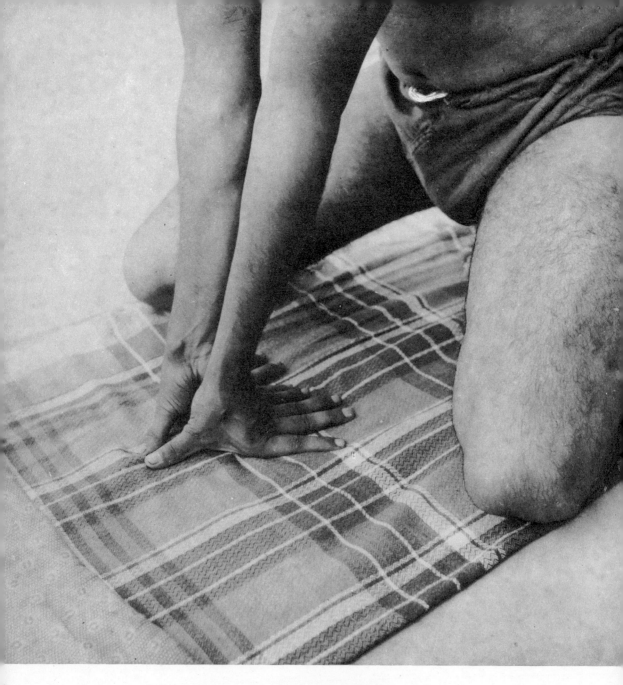

GROUP 11 – FIG. 54
Peacock Asana
Second position of hands

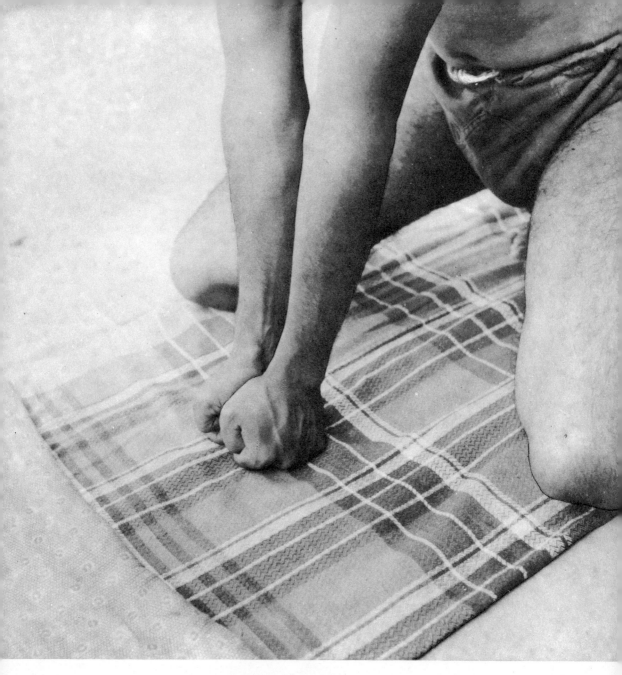

GROUP 11 – FIG. 55
Peacock Asana
Third position of hands

TWELVE IMPORTANT RECOMMENDATIONS

1. Never practise on a bed or on too soft a mattress. A single thick blanket folded in two or four should do.

2. Never breathe through the mouth during the exercises. Breathe in and out through the nose only.

3. In each degree do first the exercises which you can. Try the others but never tire yourself.

4. The relaxation posture should be adopted between each exercise for at least a minute.

5. If you particularly like an exercise, make an effort to keep it up for as long as possible, but never go beyond a quarter of an hour.

6. If you feel any pains in your limbs after the exercises or during them, rub yourself lightly with olive oil, then carry on.

7. Never begin the exercises without having obeyed the calls of nature.

8. Wear a close-fitting pair of shorts. Take off your glasses if you usually wear them.

9. Try to do breathing exercises in the stationary asanas (head stand, tree asana, complete asana, etc.).

10. After a session of asanas, rest at least ten minutes, for the energy accumulated should not be employed by the muscles, but by the internal organs and nerves. Drink a glass of milk too.

11. Concentrate your thoughts on the exercises which you are doing and don't let your mind wander.

12. Persevere. Two months are not enough. At least a year's daily practice can benefit you. The more you practise, the more you will gain.

ASANAS OF THE SECOND DEGREE

CHAPTER VI

THIS second degree of asanas is in reality only a transitional stage necessary to prepare the way for the pupil to execute more readily the harder positions at the end of this course. Generally speaking, they are only secondary poses continuing the previous ones. They are exercises tending to stretch certain muscles and sinews and prepare the body for the exercises that follow.

Yet the second and third degrees of the asanas must never lead to giving up the first-degree exercises, which are the most useful of all. The fact that you have learned to run doesn't mean that you must cease to walk.

Don't forget that you must practise regularly. Do all the movements as slowly as possible, so that they give you the maximum results. Always think intently about the exercises and the benefits which they are to bring you when you practise them. Concentration of the mind is an excellent exercise which will develop your memory and your faculties of brain and mind.

Be diligent in carrying out your exercises for controlling the breathing before and after the asanas and whenever you can do it without tiring yourself.

Don't practise if it is going to tire you or if you have some worry on your mind. The asanas should be done in good spirits, which are the outward sign of mental and physical release from tension.

Finally, if certain exercises strike you as too difficult, replace them with others which you enjoy doing more, without, however, giving up all hope. One day, to your great surprise, when your body has been limbered up by degrees, you will be able to achieve them without difficulty.

At the end we give you exercise tables which will help you to arrange your daily programme. But they are only suggestions and you must remain free to do your own self-organising.

GROUP 12

Dancing Asana *(Natarajasana)*

TECHNIQUE

1. Standing up, catch the big toe of the right foot with the right hand thrown over the shoulder, and keep your balance by raising the left arm as high as possible in the air.

2. Make the same movement with the left foot and hand. **Breathe rhythmically (Fig. 56).**

VARIATION

A development of the bow posture (Group 4), called **Purna-Dhanurasana** or **complete bow,** duplicates the dancing asana, but with both hands and legs at once, while the body rests on the stomach. The effects of this asana are the same as those produced by the dancing asana, but make themselves felt on both sides of the body at once (**Fig. 57**).

RESULTS

These movements stretch the muscles and tendons of the fore part of the body. They strengthen the rib muscles and develop general balance.

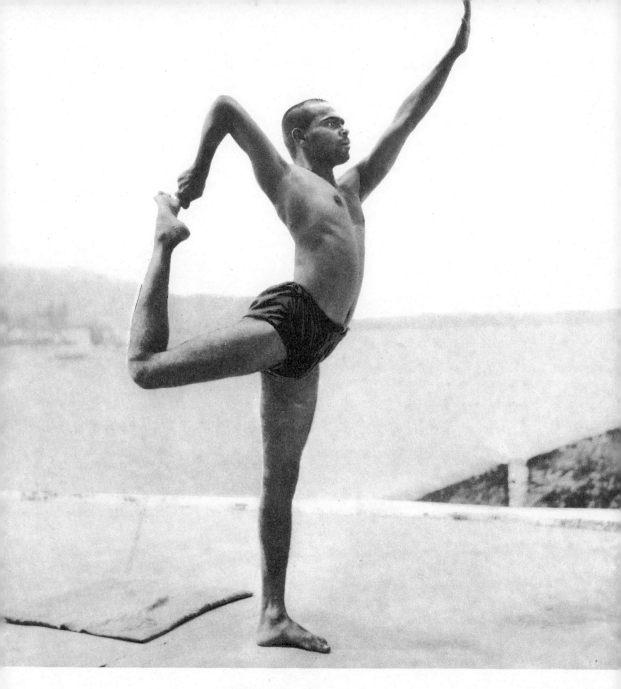

GROUP 12 – FIG. 56
Dancing Asana

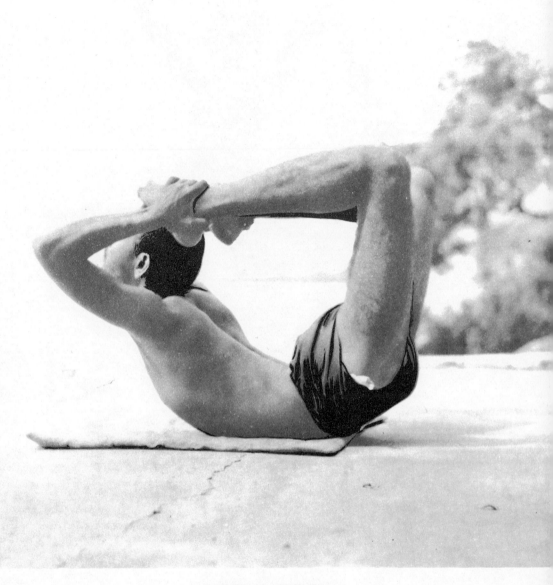

GROUP 12 – FIG. 57
Complete Bow Asana

GROUP 13

Gokarna Asana *(Gokarnasana)*

Head-and-Knees Asana *(Janusirasana)*

TECHNIQUE OF GOKARNASANA

1. Lie on your back, arms raised behind the head.

2. Put the right arm and leg at right angles to the body in a horizontal plane.

3. Catch the big toe with the hand. Keep the position for a time, then make the same movement with the opposite side of the body. **Breathe normally (Fig. 58).**

This movement stretches the adductor muscles of the thighs and shoulders.

TECHNIQUE OF JANUSIRASANA

This is in a way the **pincers asana** (Group 9), but performed with one leg, the other remaining bent at the knee at an angle of 90° with the other leg, the foot being pressed into the groin **(Fig. 59)**.

This exercise increases the suppleness of the spine and brings all the muscular force to bear on the one leg stretched out.

This exercise is recommended to be done sometimes with one leg and sometimes with the other.

G

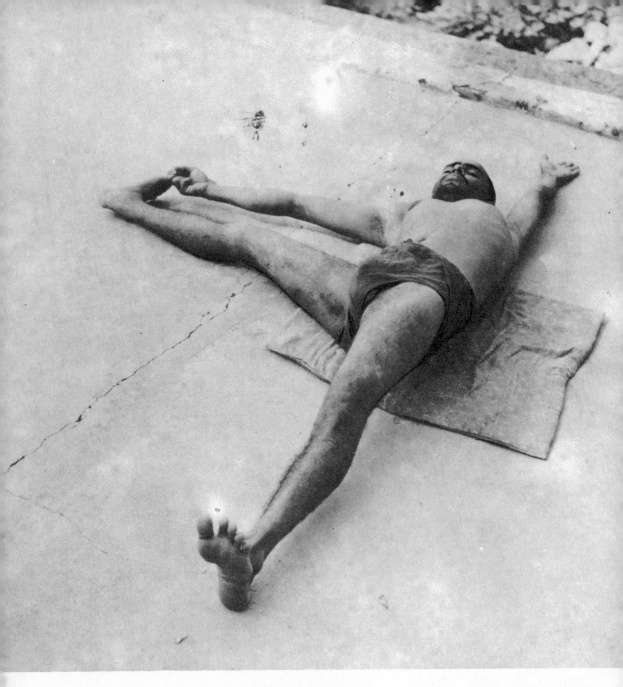

GROUP 13 – FIG. 58
Gokarna Asana

98

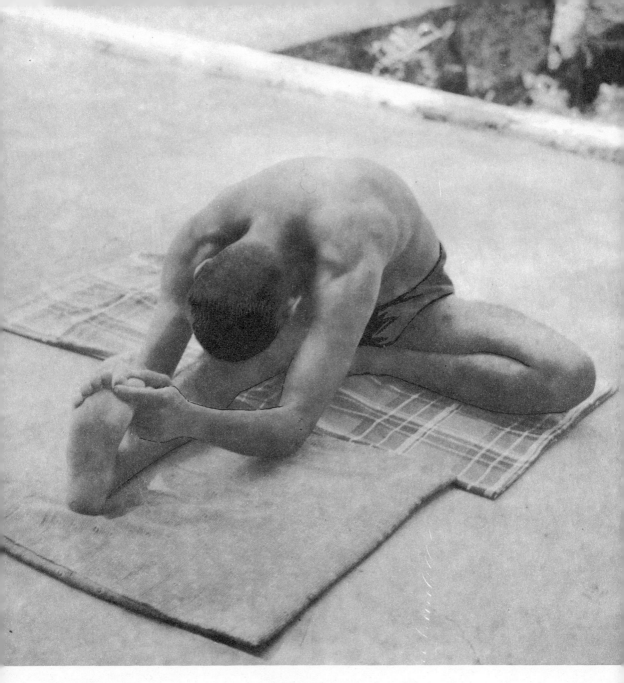

GROUP 13 – FIG. 59
Janusir Asana

GROUP 14

Hasta Padasana *(Toe-hold Asana)*

Kurmasana *(Tortoise Asana)*

These two exercises of increasing difficulty make the spinal column more flexible, strengthen the neck muscles, massage the thyroid gland and increase the chest capacity. The functions of digestion are speeded up.

HASTA-PADASANA

1. Sit on the blanket, the legs as far apart as possible.

2. Bend your body forward to touch the ground with your forehead.

3. Grasp the toes with the hands (**Fig. 60**). **Breathe slowly and deeply.**

KURMASANA (The Tortoise)

Do the preceding exercise, but instead of grasping the toes with the hands pass the arms back under the thighs. **Breathe gently**, then return to the extended position and rest (**Fig. 61**).

RESULTS

Stretching of the spinal column and massage of the major sympathetic and the thyroid. Influx of blood to the throat. The whole nervous system is rejuvenated.

100

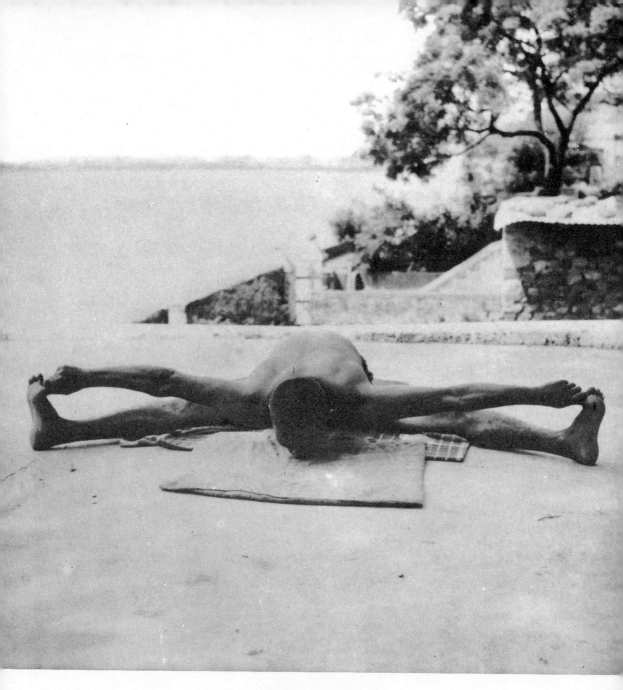

GROUP 14 – FIG. 60
Toe-hold Asana

101

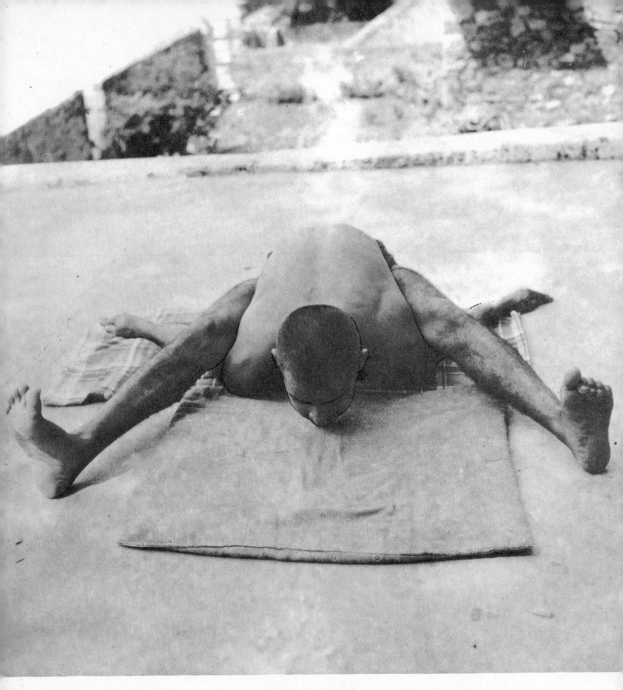

GROUP 14 – FIG. 61
Tortoise Asana

ASANAS OF REST, STILLNESS AND MENTAL BALANCE

These asanas are not recommended to beginners. They are in general utilised for spiritual ends and for meditation. They are a rest only for those who have long been used to them.

They are:

The Hero Asana;

The Adept Asana;

The Prosperity Asana;

The Tiptoe Asana.

You can try to perform them, but they are hardly useful to those who do not practise meditation.

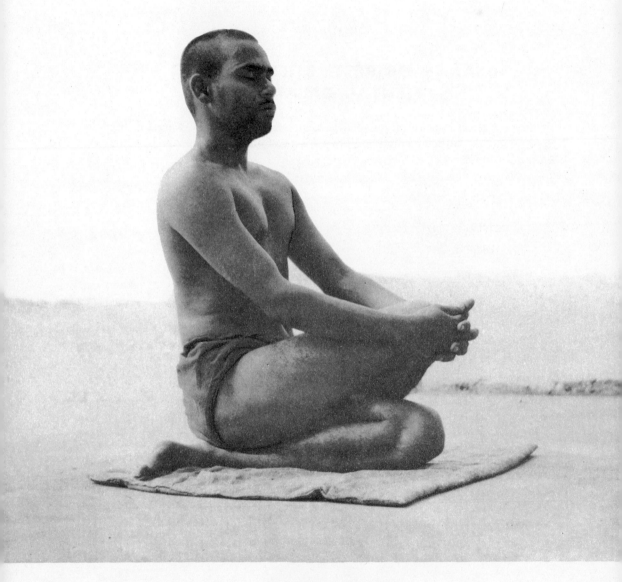

GROUP 15 – FIG. 62

Hero Asana *(Virasana)*

1. Sit on one heel.
2. Cross the free leg over the opposite thigh.
3. Cross the hands with fingers interlocked on the knee. Hold the head and shoulders straight.

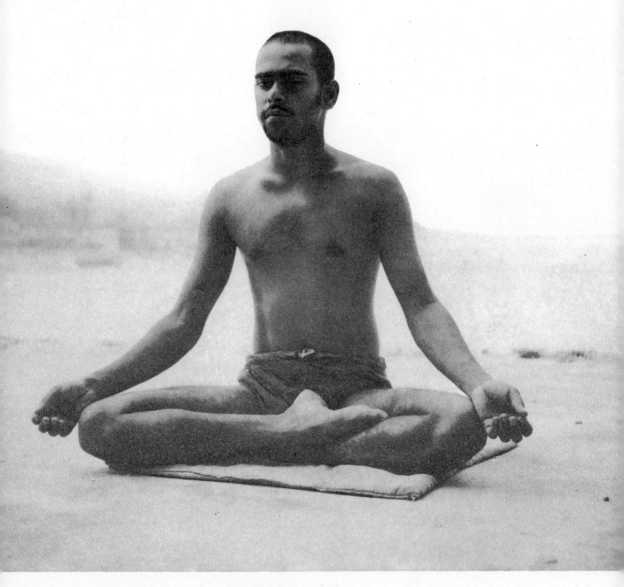

GROUP 15 – FIG. 63
Adept Asana *(Sidasana)*

1. Sit cross-legged.
2. Insert the toes of one foot between the thigh and calf of the opposite leg. Hold the body and head straight.

105

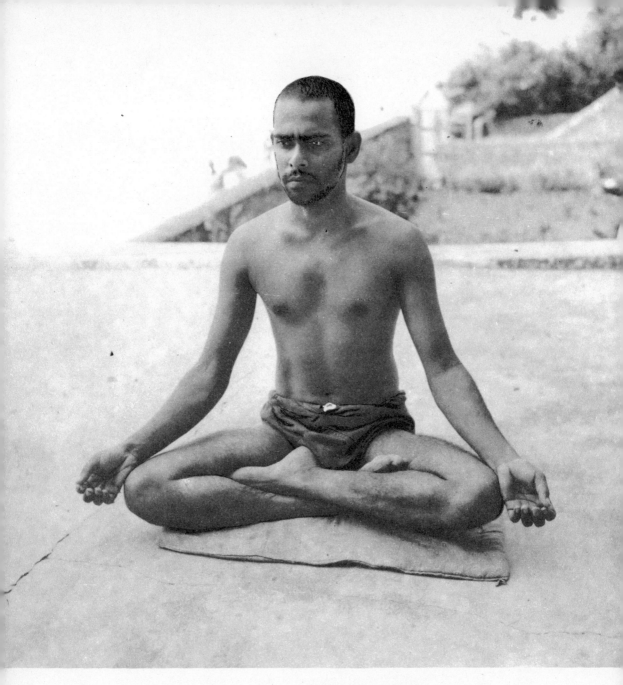

GROUP 15 – FIG. 64
Prosperity Asana (*Svastikasana*)

1. Adopt the preceding pose.
2. Insert the toes of each foot between the thigh and calf of the opposite leg.

106

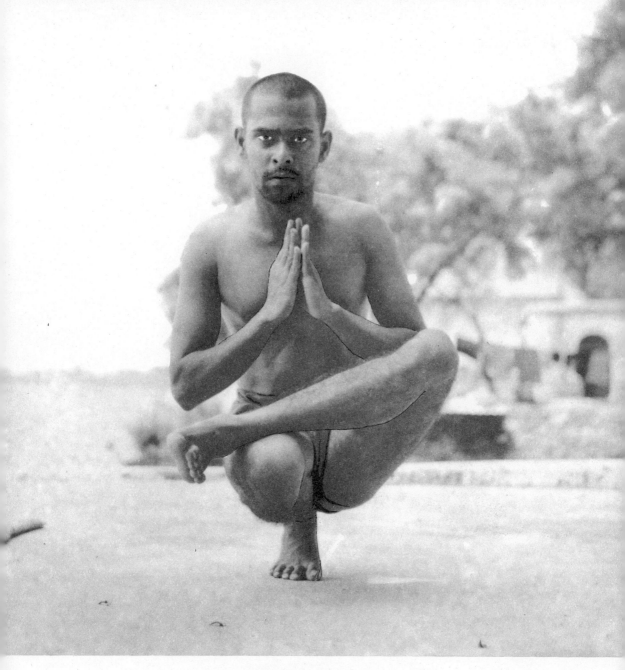

GROUP 15 – FIG. 65
Tiptoe Asana *(Padangushtasana)*

1. Sit on tiptoe.
2. Cross one leg over the other.
3. When balance is attained, put the hands together at chest height. Keep absolutely still, fixing the gaze on the hands as long as possible, **while you breathe slowly and deeply.** This last mentioned posture develops to the highest degree the possibilities of mental concentration and singleness of thought as well as physical balance.

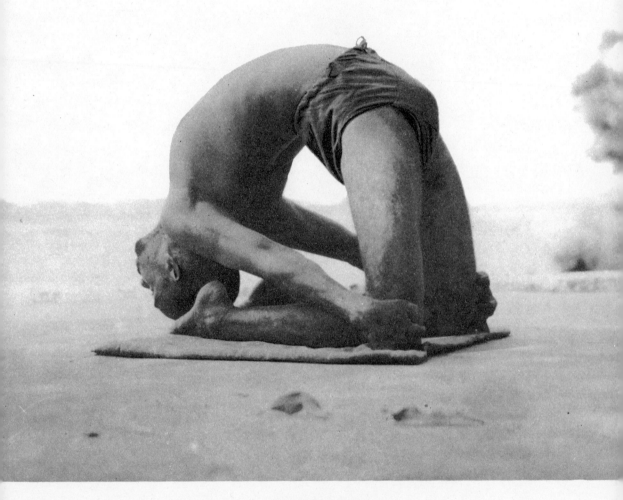

GROUP 16 – FIG. 66
Purna-Supta-Vajrasana

The asanas of this group are but simple variants or completions of the diamond pose (Group 8), the locust asana (Group 6) and the cobra posture (Group 5), and have the same effects as these. They increase, however, the flexibility of the body and considerably develop the thoracic cage.

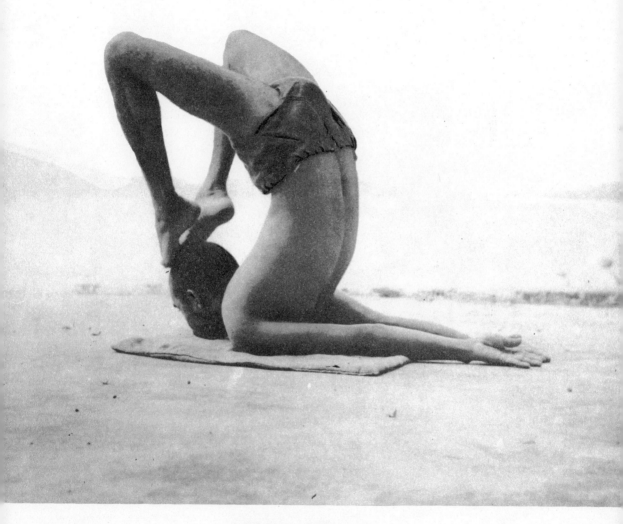

GROUP 16 – FIG. 67
Viparita-Halasana

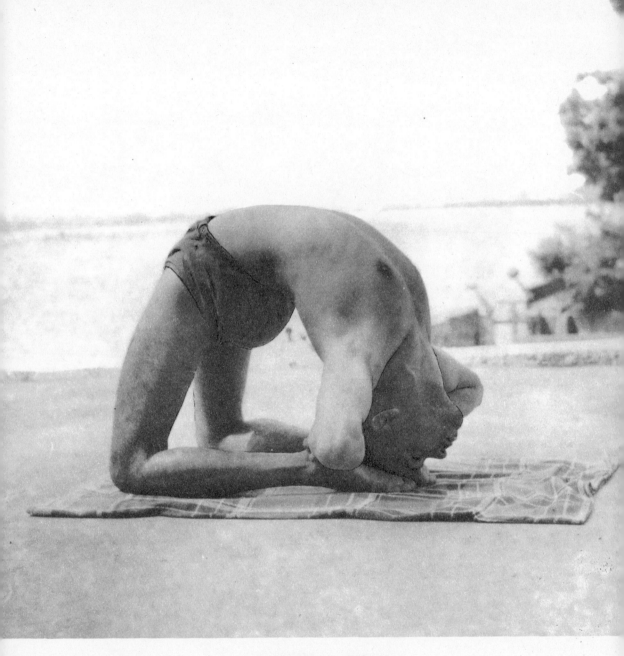

GROUP 16 – FIG. 68
Purna-Supta-Vajrasana

110

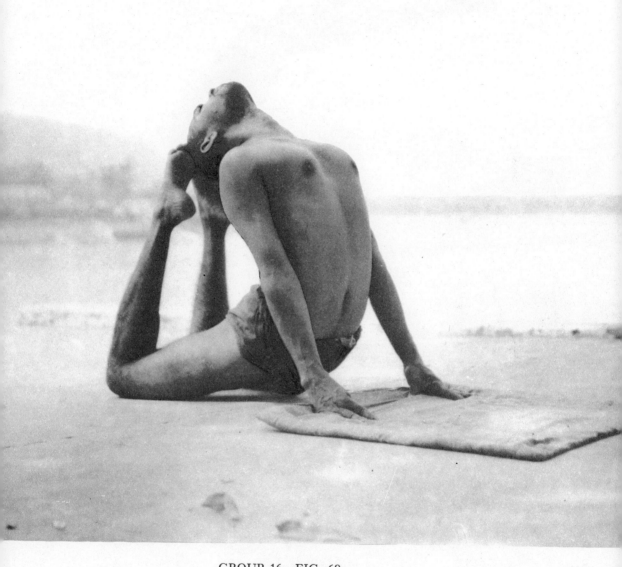

GROUP 16 – FIG. 69
Padasirshasana

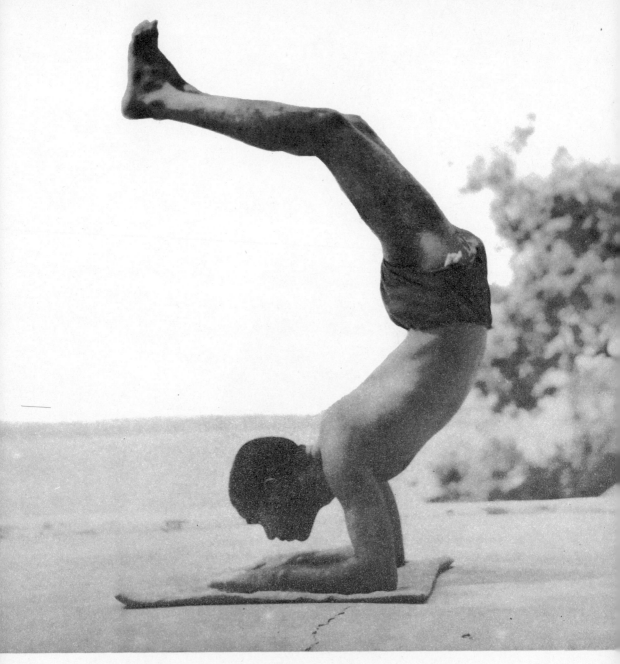

GROUP 17 – FIG. 70
Half-Scorpion Asana (*Ardha-Vrichikasana*)

These asanas develop balance and strengthen the arm, rib and loin muscles. In addition they give the same results as the head stand.

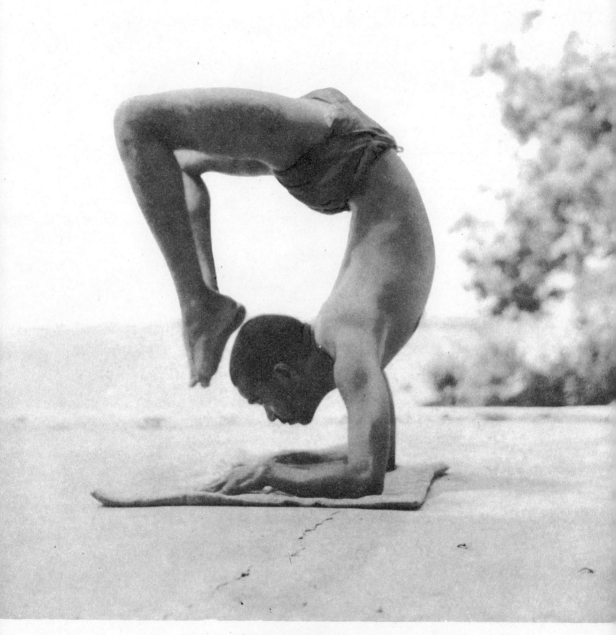

GROUP 17 – FIG. 71

Scorpion Asana *(Vrichikasana)*

These two asanas, the half-scorpion and the scorpion, are a development of the head stand (Group 1). But in them the head no longer touches the ground and the body is supported only by the forearms and hands.

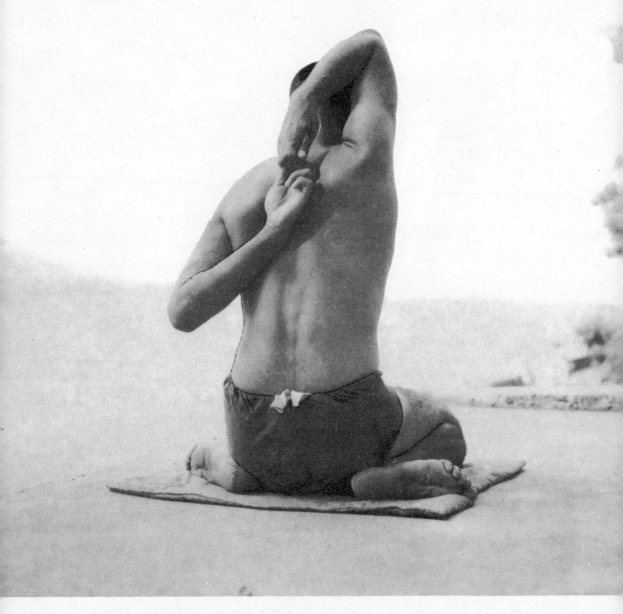

GROUP 18 – FIG. 72
Cow's-head Asana *(Gomukhasana)*

This asana develops the trapezoidal muscles and increases the capacity of the thoracic cage. It can be practised sitting or standing. It consists simply in joining the hands behind the back by passing one arm over the shoulder.

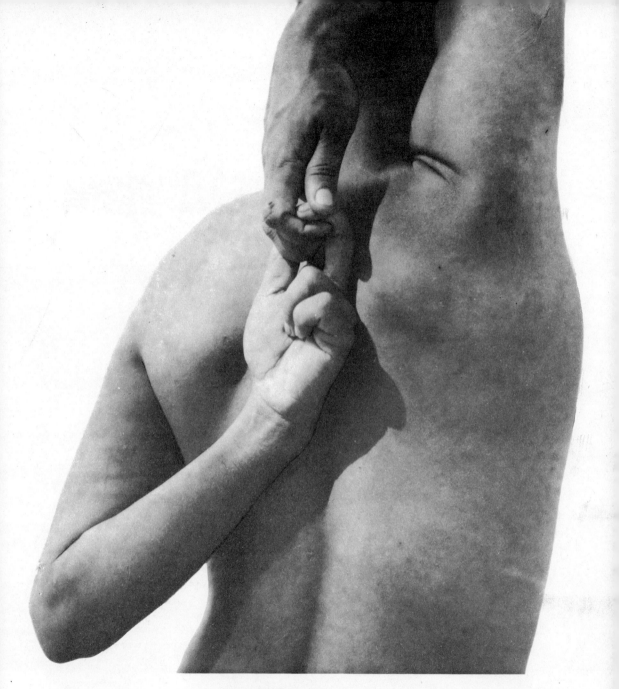

GROUP 18 – FIG. 73

Cow's-head Asana

Detail of the hands. Make this join with left and right hands alternately, and pull on the fingers as hard as possible.

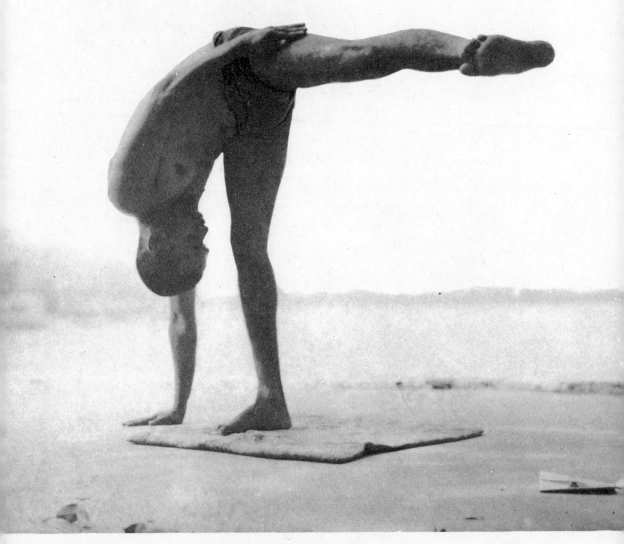

GROUP 19 – FIG 74
One-legged Asana *(Ekapadahastasana)*

TECHNIQUE.—

1. Standing with feet together, touch the ground in front of the feet with the palms of the hands, **breathing out.**

2. Raise one leg at right angles to the side and lay the corresponding arm along the body. Maintain the balance.

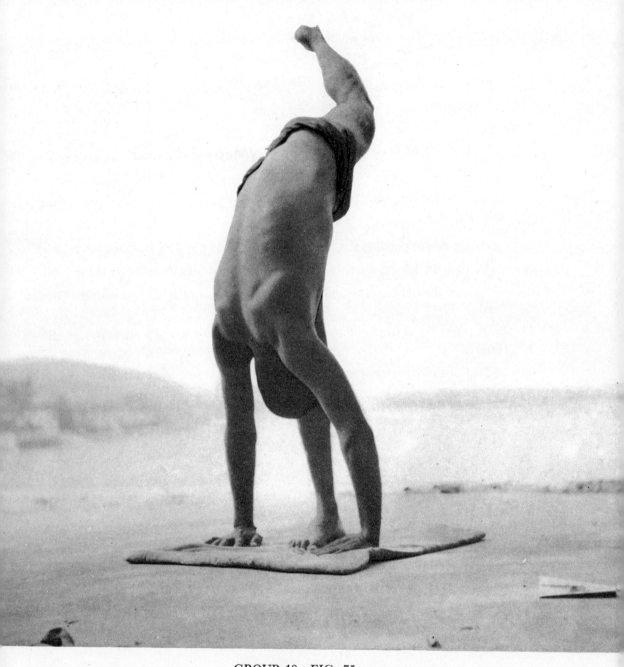

GROUP 19 – FIG. 75

One-legged Asana

VARIATION. Perform the same movement keeping both hands on the ground and throwing one leg as high as possible to the rear in line with the body.

RESULTS. The thigh and abdominal muscles are strengthened and expanded.

GROUP 20

Matsyendra Asanas *(Matsyendrasana)*

TECHNIQUE

1. Sit down, bending the right leg so that the right heel is under the crutch.

2. Pass the left leg over the right thigh and plant the foot flat on the ground.

3. Pass the right arm behind the left knee and grasp the left foot with the right hand.

4. Turn the entire body and the head towards the left side. **Breathe gently (Fig. 76).**

Repeat this movement to the right.

VARIATIONS

Do the same exercise catching the right leg with the right hand behind the body. Repeat with the left hand and leg (**Figs. 77, 78**).

Instead of sitting on your heel, bend your leg completely to wedge your foot in the groin of the opposite leg, so that you are sitting on your thigh. The movement of the body and arms remains the same (**Fig. 79**).

RESULTS

By giving the body a side-twist, the spinal column is made supple laterally, the tracts of the major sympathetic toned up, and the muscles of the back massaged. This asana cures nervous troubles in general and, by massaging the abdominal organs, eliminates the poisons due to the processes of digestion.

118

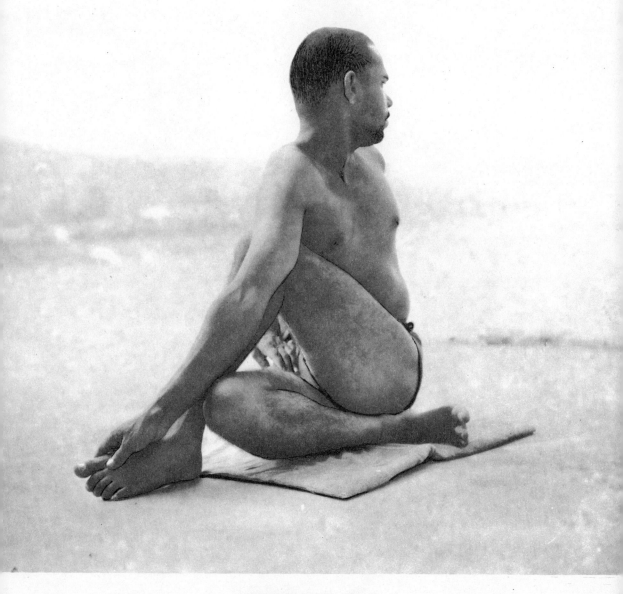

GROUP 20 – FIG. 76

Matsyendra Asana

By giving the body a side-twist, the spinal column is made supple laterally, the tracts of the major sympathetic toned up, and the muscles of the back massaged. This asana cures nervous troubles in general and, by massaging the abdominal organs, eliminates the poisons due to the processes of digestion.

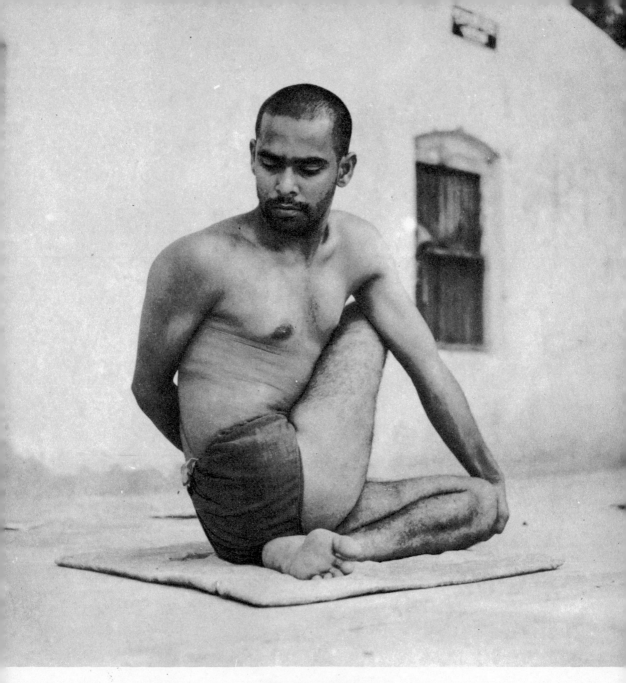

GROUP 20 – FIG. 77
Matsyendra Asana
Variation

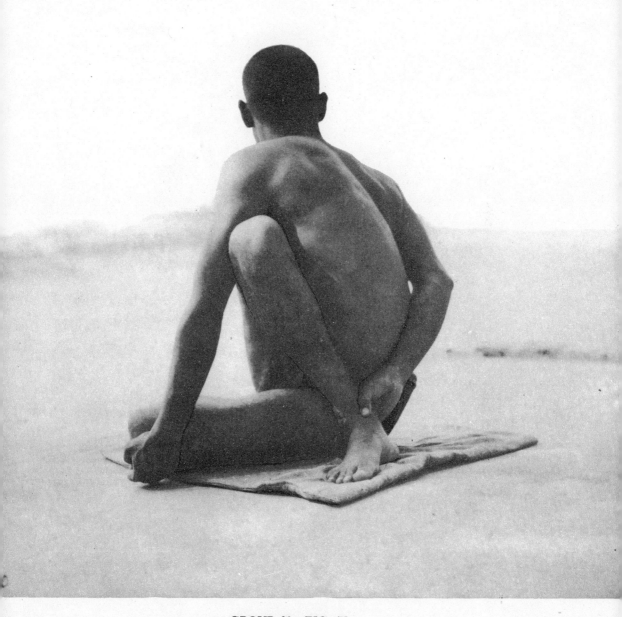

GROUP 20 – FIG. 78
Matsyendra Asana
Variation

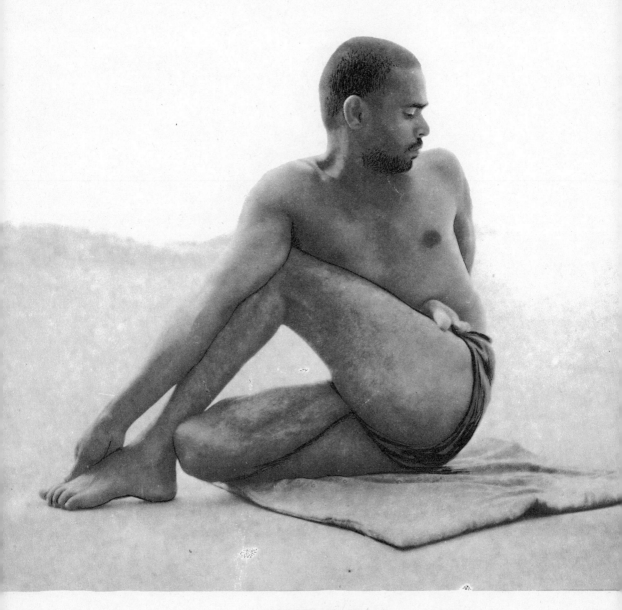

GROUP 20 – FIG. 79
Matsyendra Asana
Variation

122

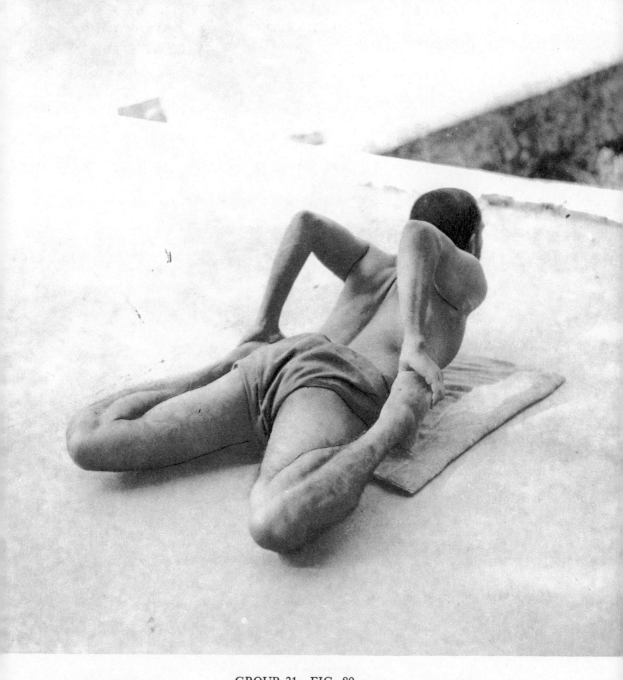

GROUP 21 – FIG. 80

Bird Asana (*Bhegasana*)

Lying on the stomach, grasp your feet with the hands and, throwing the elbows back, press down on the feet as you hold the body and head up as high as you can. **Breathe in and out rhythmically.**

RESULTS. The asanas of Group 21 aim at developing the greatest possible flexibility, making supple and expanding the muscles of legs, abdomen, arms and feet.

123

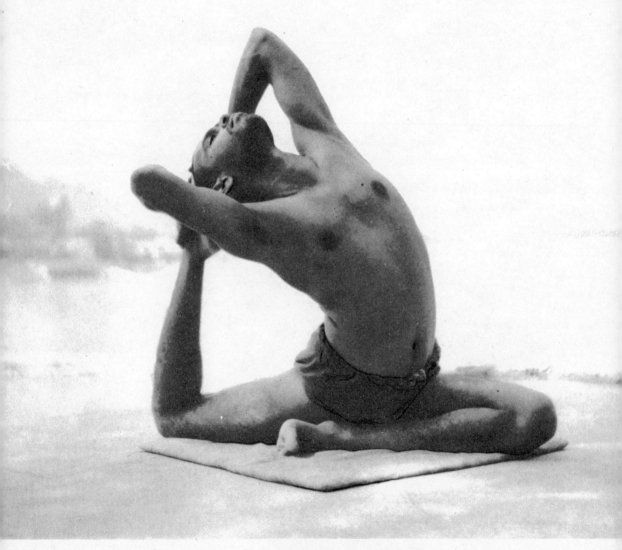

GROUP 21 – FIG. 81
Bird's-head Asana *(Kapodasana)*

Sit with one leg doubled under the body and the other thrown backwards. Catch the foot of the leg behind with both your hands raised above the head and pull to bring the foot in contact with the head. **Inhale and hold the breath.**

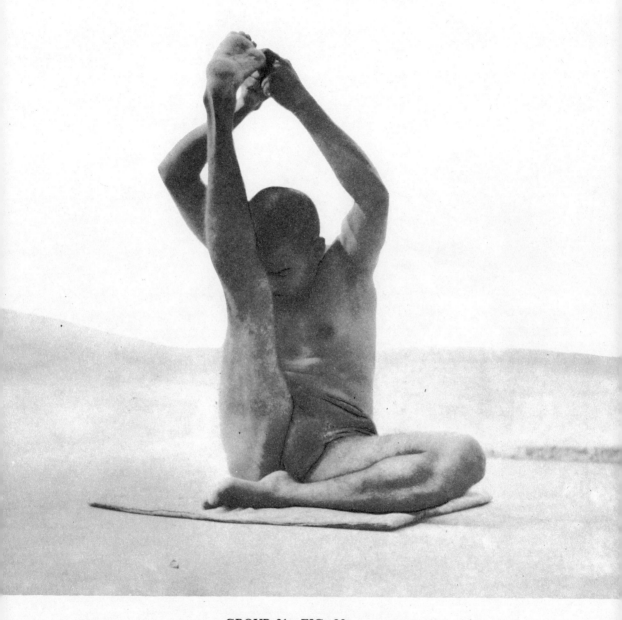

GROUP 21 – FIG. 82
Vertical Janusir Asana *(Jauusirasana)*

Sit in the disciple posture (Group 8). Then raise the extended leg vertically by hooking the hands on to the toes. The head should touch the knee, the other leg remaining doubled. Keep this position while you **breathe gently (Fig. 82).**

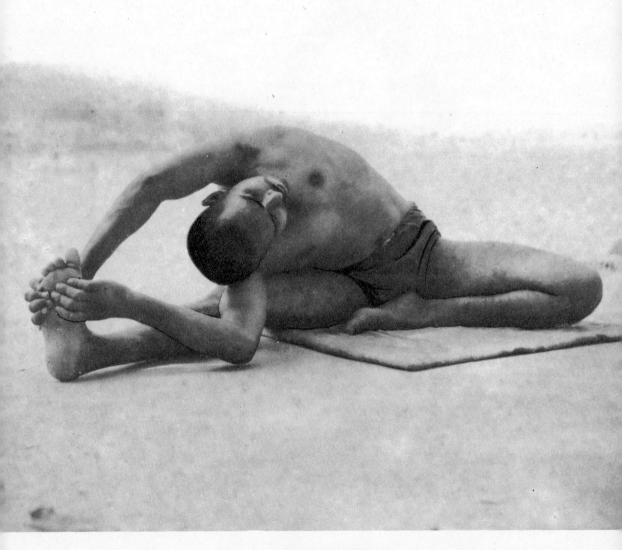

GROUP 21 – FIG. 83
Janusir Asana

VARIANT. Seated in the disciple position (Group 8), lean forward and catch the toes of the extended leg. At the same time give the body a half-turn, one of the elbows touching the ground (**Fig. 83**).

ASANAS OF THE THIRD DEGREE

CHAPTER VII

THE postures or asanas which form this third degree are extremely difficult to accomplish. Only those persons with plenty of training and great suppleness, natural or acquired, will be able to achieve them rapidly. They are almost all postures of stability. It is necessary, when practising them, to keep the position as long as possible. These asanas give less immediate benefit than those of the first degree, which are the most perfect.

So we will describe them only in brief. The beginner will not require to practise them before at least a year's regular training with the other asanas. An ill-prepared body and a non-stabilised mind would not be able to get any benefit from them, and certain physical or mental disorders might crop up which he would be hard put to it to master.

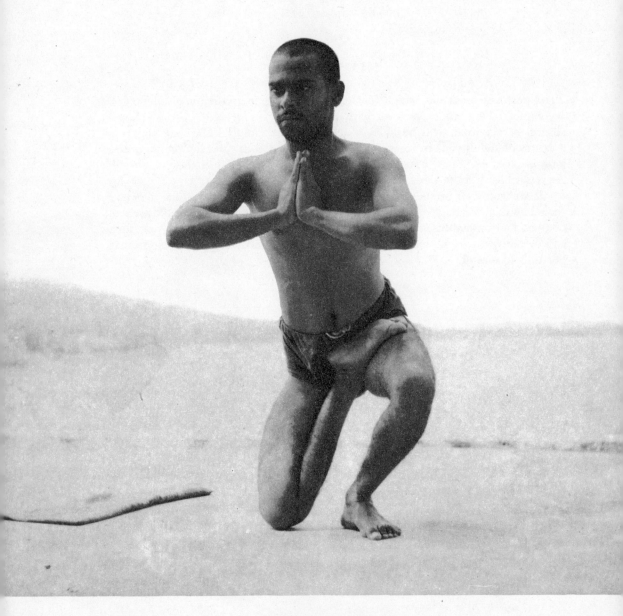

GROUP 22 – FIG. 84
Half-leg Asana *(Vatyanasana)*

This is a stable posture of balance. Stand up slowly and then return to the position. The whole strength is thus concentrated in a single leg at a time. Make the same movement changing legs each time.

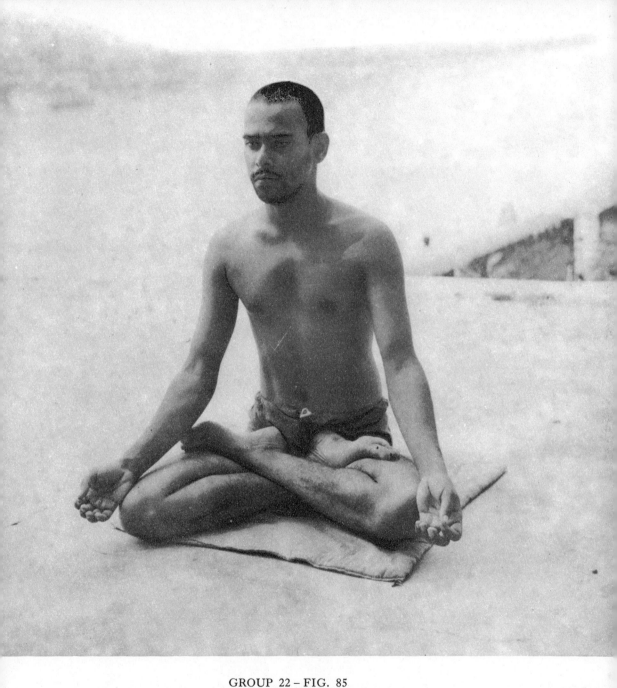

GROUP 22 – FIG. 85
Lotus Asana *(Padmasana)*

This sitting position is very comfortable to adopt for orientals, who are used to it from their childhood. But for a westerner it is very difficult to take up and especially to hold. Put the feet in position on the thighs with the help of the hands. This posture, assumed after meals, aids digestion. It relieves attacks of rheumatism and invigorates the nerves of the legs and thighs.

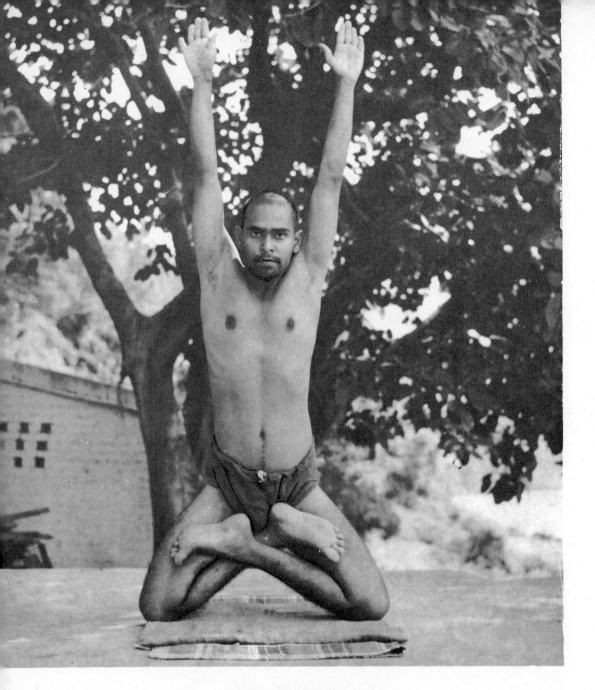

GROUP 23 – FIG. 86

Mountain Asana *(Parbatasana)*

This posture derives directly from the previous one. It lengthens all the thigh and trunk muscles and develops maximum balance and mental concentration.

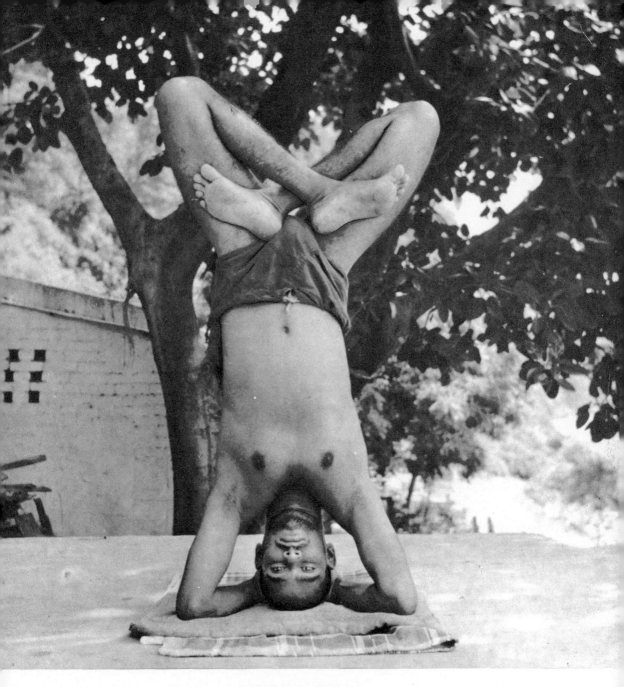

GROUP 23 – FIG. 87
Inverted Lotus Asana *(Urdwa-Padmasana)*

This asana is similar to the head stand (Group 1), but with the legs in the lotus posture. It has the same results as the head stand, of which it is simply a variation.

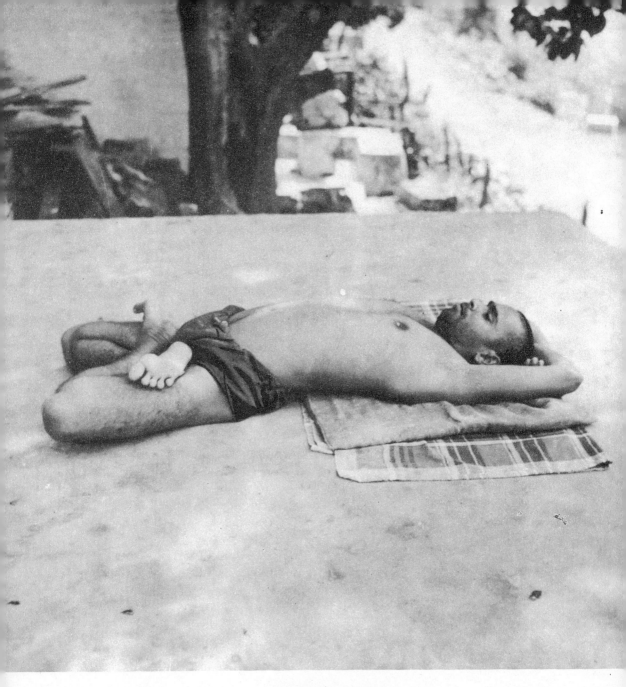

GROUP 24 – FIG. 88
Fish Asana (*Matsyasana*)

Lie flat on your back in the lotus posture and cross the hands behind the head. In this position the body can float with ease in water without risk of drowning. This asana cures muscular and nervous complaints of the neck and cervical region. It feeds the thyroid and parathyroid and develops the chest and back.

132

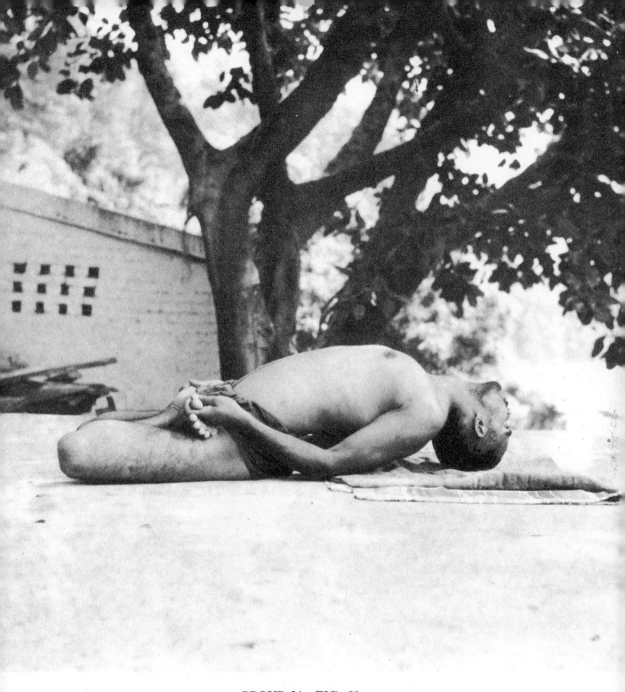

GROUP 24 – FIG. 89
Fish Asana

VARIATION. A variant of this position consists in grasping the toes with the hands and arching the body so that it no longer rests on the ground except at the thighs, buttocks and head. The previous effects are intensified.

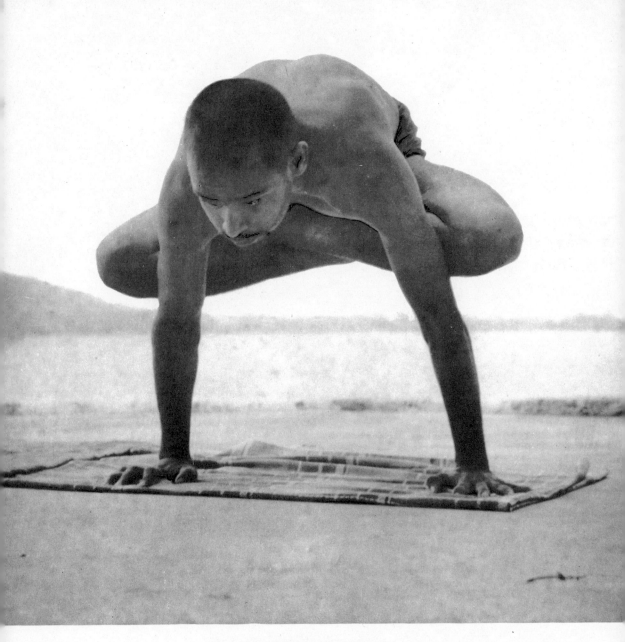

GROUP 25 – FIG. 90
Raised Lotus Asana (*Uttitha-Padmasana*)

Sit in the lotus posture, placing the hands in front of you on the ground. Then, leaning forward, raise the thighs slowly in the air, the legs resting on the arms. This posture develops the muscles and nerves of the hands, arms and shoulders and strengthens the abdominal walls.

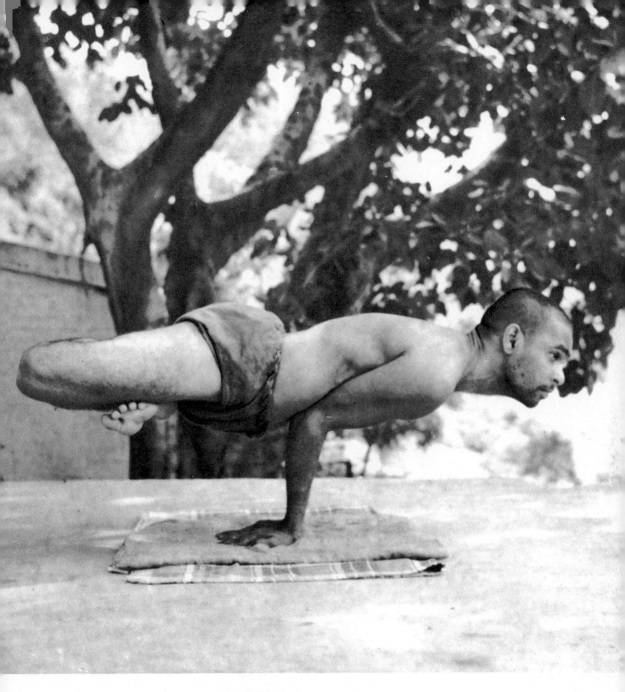

GROUP 25 – FIG. 91

Balance Asana (Lolasana)

This is only a variation of the peacock asana (Group 11) with the feet in the lotus
position. The results obtained are identical.

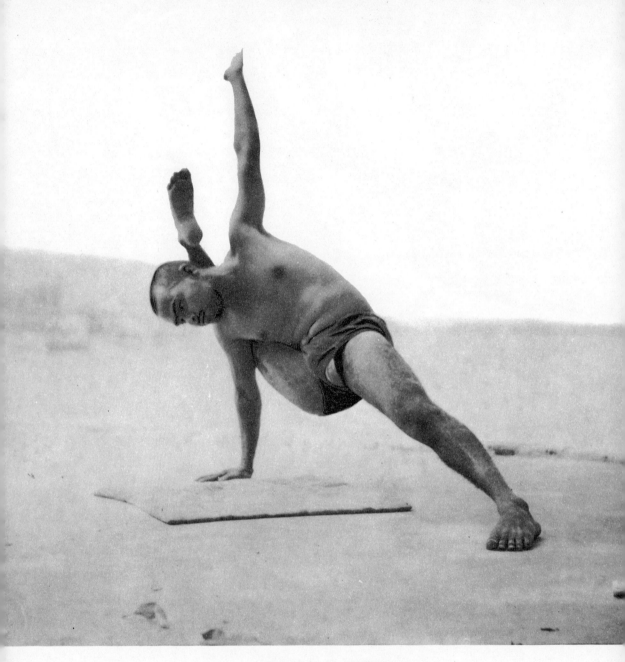

GROUP 26 – FIG. 92
Krishna Asana (*Krishnasana*)

One leg is passed over the head and wedged against the nape of the neck. The balance is kept on the other leg and the opposite arm.

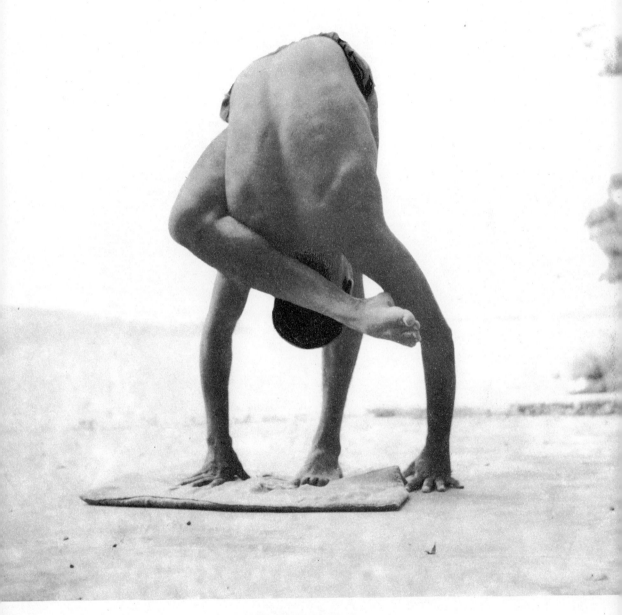

GROUP 26 – FIG. 93
Single-footed Asana *(Ekapadahastasana)*

One leg is passed over the head and wedged against the nape of the neck. Lean forward and touch the ground with both your hands, the other leg remaining straight.

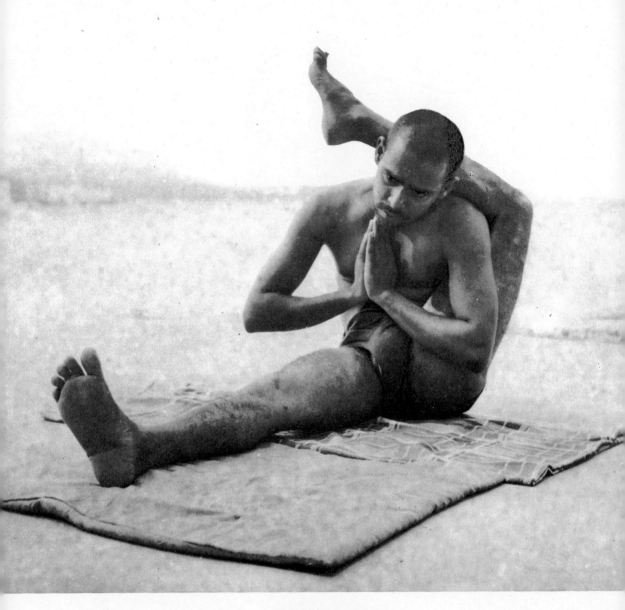

GROUP 26 – FIG. 94
Single-footed Asana

VARIATION. A variant of this asana consists in sitting in this position and putting the hands together on the chest.

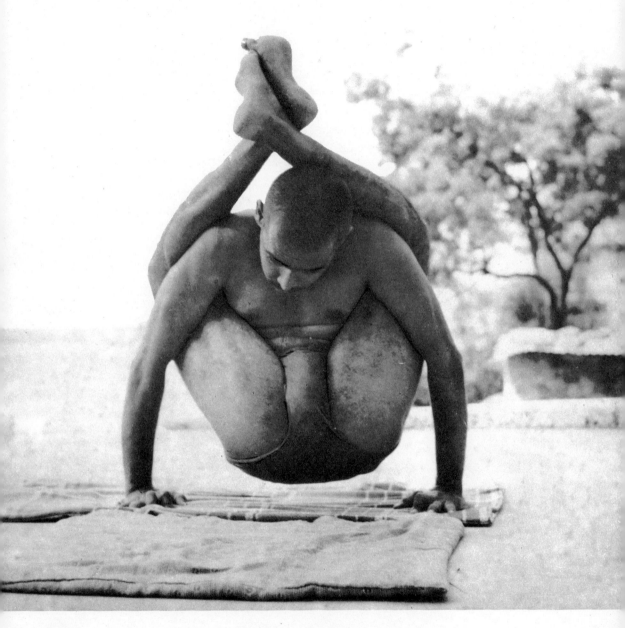

GROUP 26 – FIG. 95

Upright Tortoise Asana *(Uttitha-Kurmasana)*

After passing both legs over the head and crossing them at the back of the neck, try to keep your balance on the hands only.

The asanas of Group 26 are all intended to massage the intestinal organs and promote the secretions of the liver, bile and pancreas.

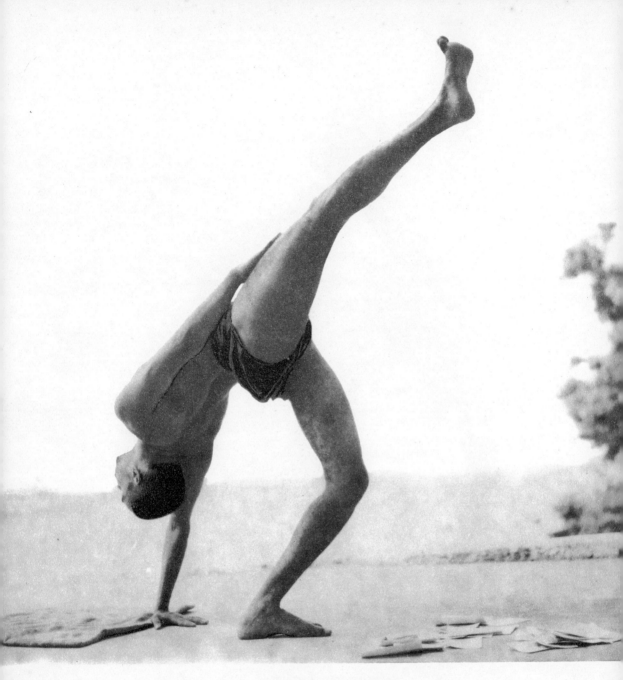

GROUP 27 – FIG. 96
Half-wheel Asana (*Ardha-Chakrasana*)

After performing the wheel asana (Group 3), lift one leg as high as possible while keeping the corresponding arm close to the side of the body. This asana has the same effects as the corresponding one in Group 3, of which it is only a variation.

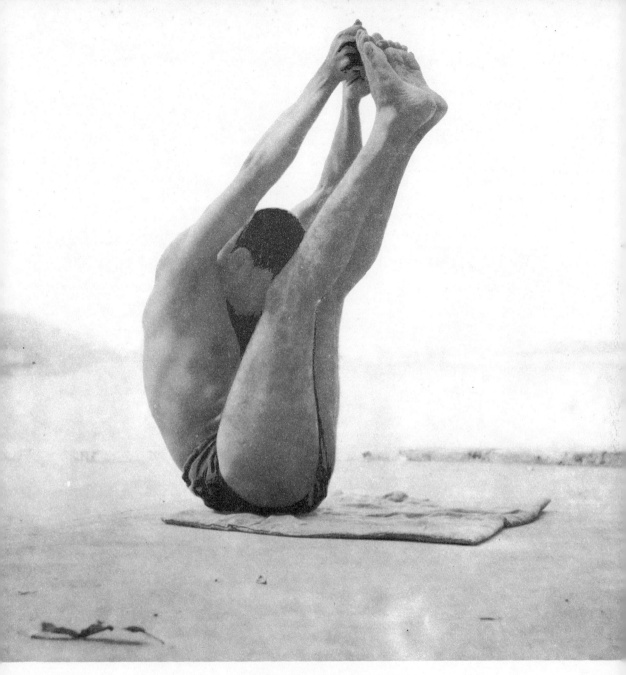

GROUP 27 – FIG. 97
Raised Pincers Asana (*Urdwa-Paschimottanasana*)

This is the pincers asana (Group 9) performed with the legs in the air, the body being supported only on the buttocks.

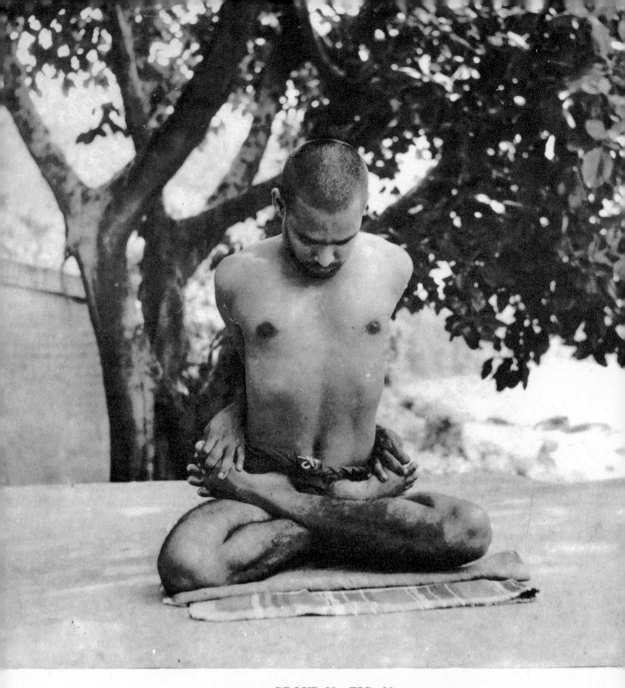

GROUP 28 – FIG. 98
Locked Lotus Asana *(Baddha Padmasana)*

Sitting in the lotus position, cross the arms behind the back and catch the toes with the hands. This asana considerably develops the thoracic cage.

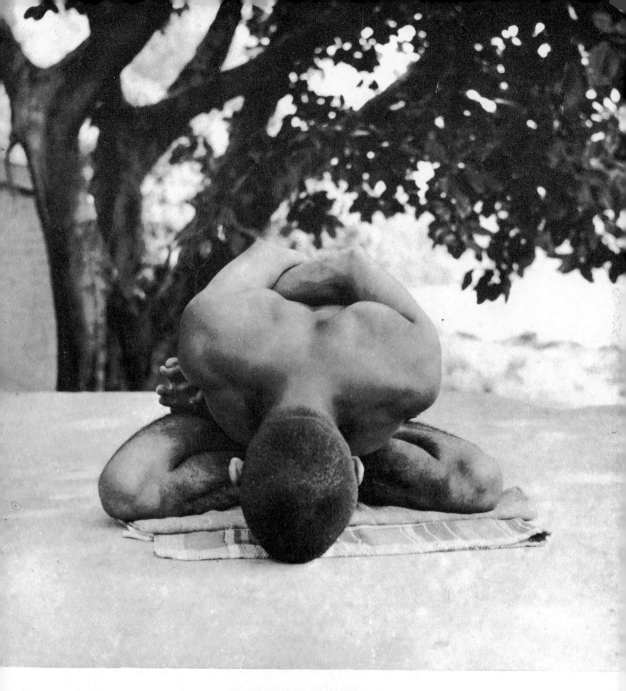

GROUP 28 – FIG. 99
Yoga Seal *(Yoga-Mudra)*

Sitting in the previous position, touch the ground in front of you with the forehead. This latter position is very dangerous to keep up for long and it will be in the interest of students not to stay in it.

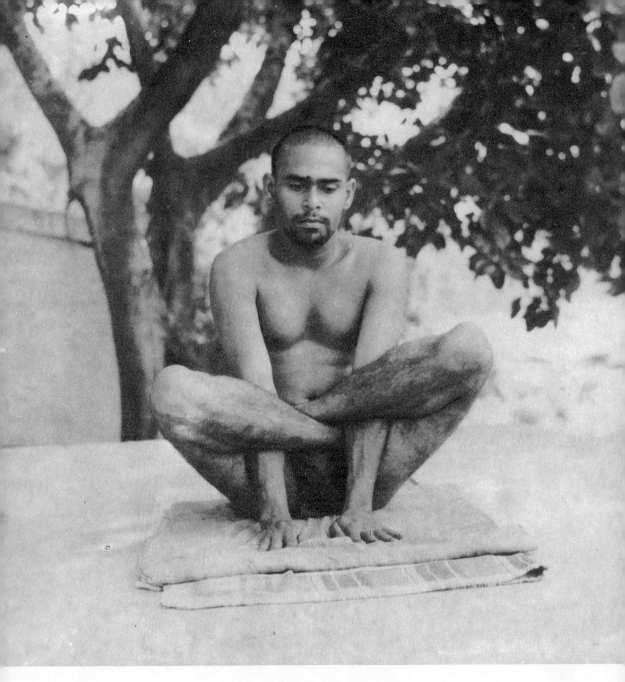

GROUP 29 – FIG. 100
Cock Asana *(Kukkutasana)*
Starting position

Sitting in the lotus posture, pass the arms between the calves and the thighs and raise the body.

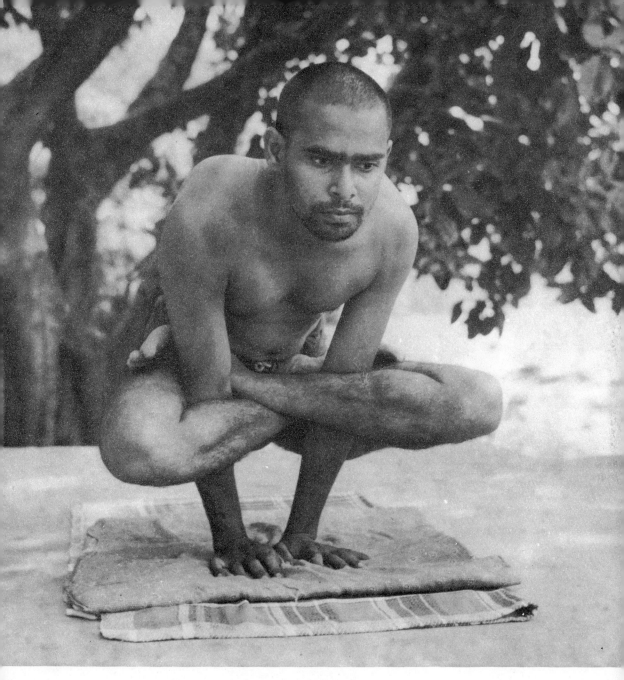

GROUP 29 – FIG. 101
Cock Asana
Keeping the balance develops the arm and neck muscles.

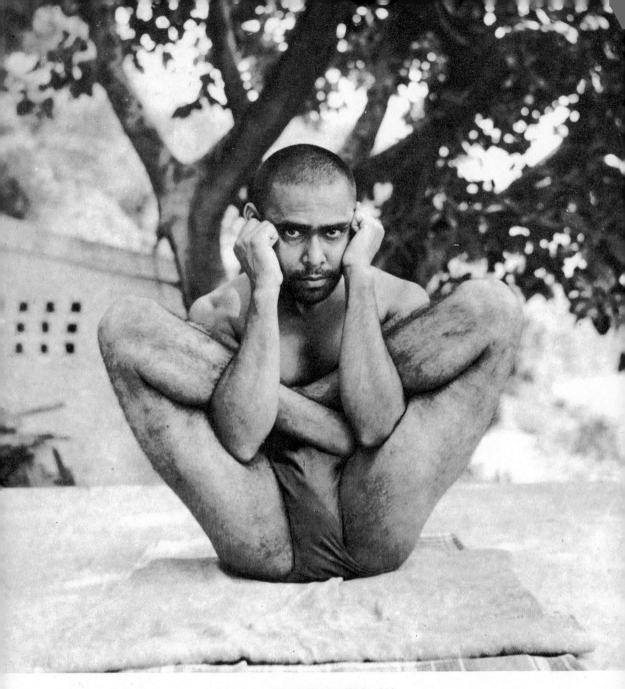

GROUP 29 – FIG. 102
Foetus Asana (*Garbhasana*)

This is the same movement as before, but, instead of raising the body, bring the arms towards your face and catch the ears with the hands, balancing on the buttocks. This asana looks like a knot. Almost all the functions of the body are impeded. So you must never stay long in this position. It is an asana which slows up the vital functions.

GROUP 30

Nauli

This last group belongs to a special category, the **Kriyas** or internal cleansing exercises. We have, however, included them in the asanas, for these exercises are much more useful for strengthening the vital organs by internal massage than for purifying them, that is to say, cleansing them.

This combination of movements, conditioned essentially by the will, cures most stomach and intestinal disorders almost instantly. Don't forget that you must perform it only for a very short period each time and with the lungs completely emptied.

In practice **Nauli** is for almost daily use and it is of very great value. Never do it after a meal. Relax after this exercise and drink a large glass of pure water.

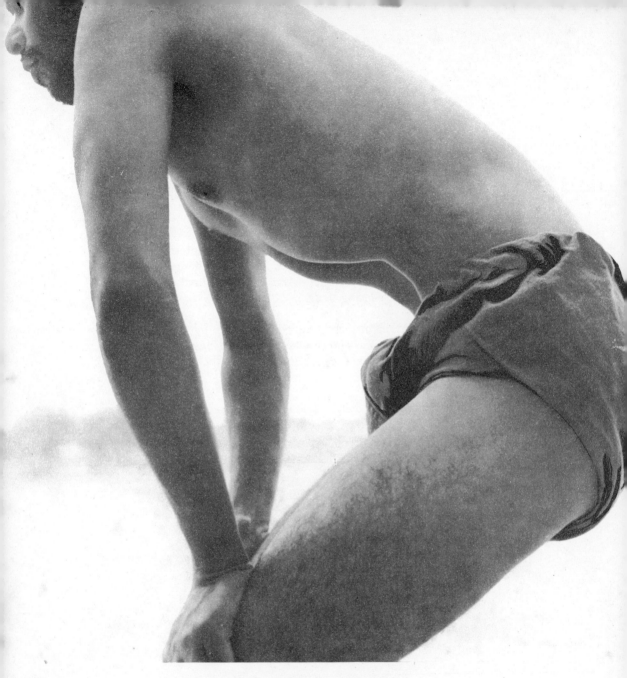

GROUP 30 – FIG. 103

Uddiyana Bandha

1. Bend the body slightly forward and rest both hands on the thighs. **Empty your lungs completely.** Then contract your abdominal muscles and bring the abdominal wall in close proximity to the spinal column. The stomach thus presents a deep pit. You will not be able to pass to the next stage without having made a complete success of this one.

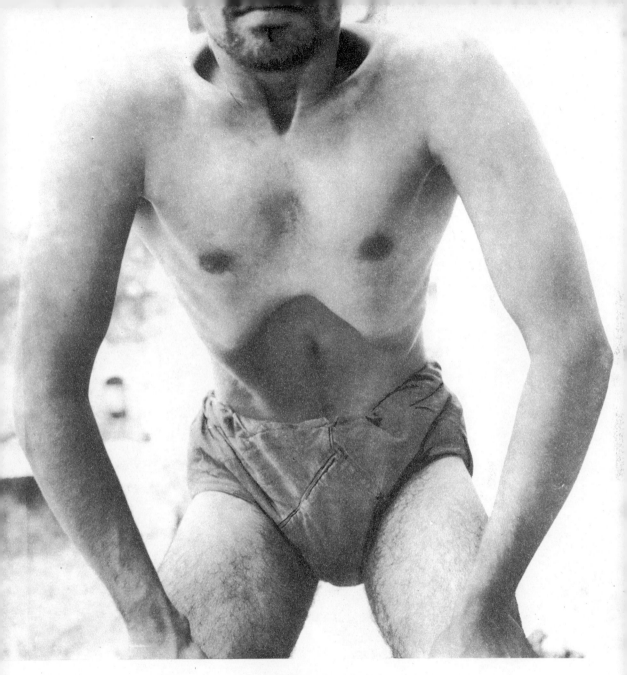

GROUP 30 – FIG. 104
Uddiyana Bandha
Front

2. Having fully accomplished this position, contract only the sides of the abdomen, so as
   to leave it hollow in the centre.

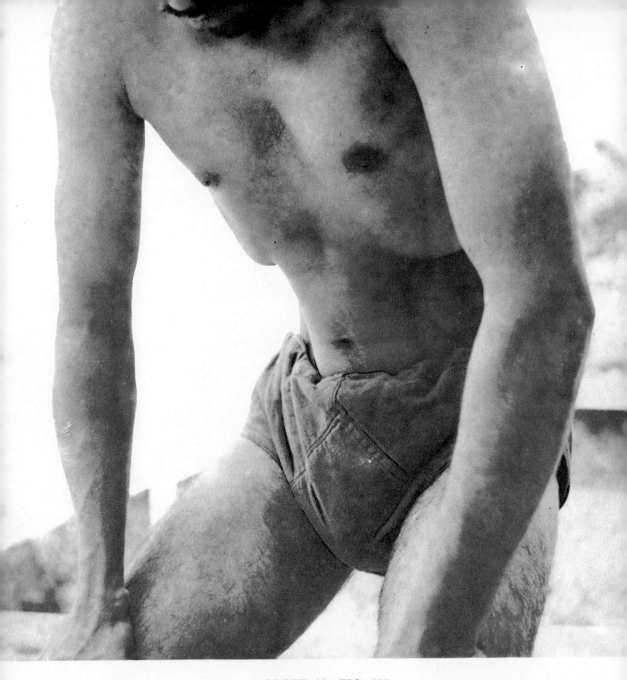

GROUP 30 – FIG. 105
Madyama Nauli

3. Do the opposite and contract all the centre muscles to form a vertical column in the middle of the abdomen.

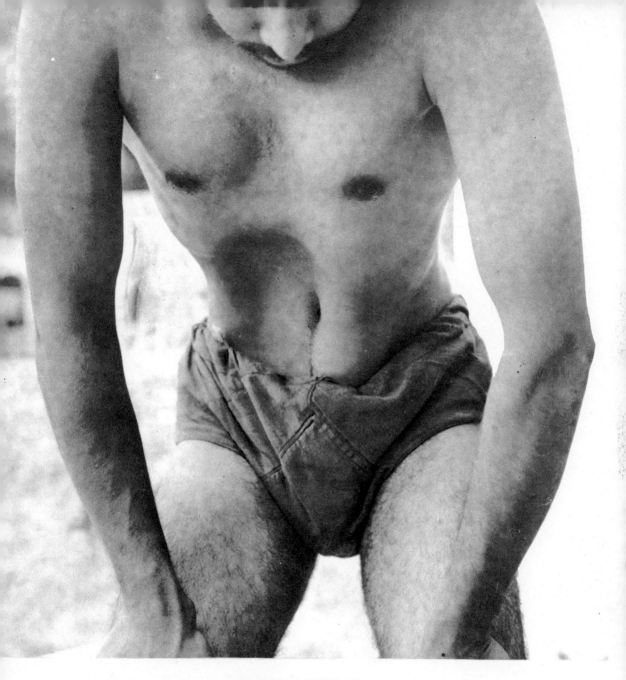

GROUP 30 – FIG. 106
Dakshina Nauli

4. Relax your muscles, then contract only those of the right side, pressing on the right thigh with the hand to give yourself more force.

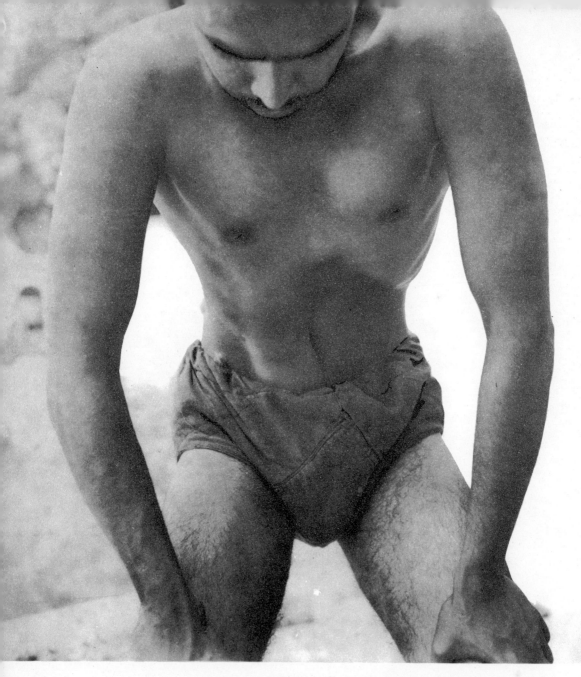

GROUP 30 – FIG. 107
Vamana Nauli

5. Relax your muscles and do the same thing with the left side of the abdomen. When you have made a success of the preceding exercises, do them again one after the other in a horizontal turning movement, slowly at first, then quickening it up. A machine will then seem to be at work in the stomach.

T R A I N I N G   T A B L E S

CHAPTER VIII

THESE tables are valid for men, women and children. They will guide you in setting up your own daily training programme. It is up to you to adopt them as we offer you them or modify them according to your aptitudes, interest and the time at your disposal.

First Stage

1. Salute to the Sun . . . . . 3 times
2. Relaxation . . . .
3. Head Stand (Group 1). . . . . 30 seconds
4. Relaxation . . . .
5. Complete Asana (Group 2) . . . . 1 minute
6. Relaxation . . . .
7. Salute to the Sun . . . . . 3 times
8. Breath-control . . . . . . 2 minutes

Total time: 8–10 minutes.

This first stage is to be recommended for younger children and for persons whose state of health does not allow them to make very sustained efforts. It is also suitable for persons with little time to spare.

It is wise to practise this training for three months before embarking on the following:

Second Stage

1. Salute to the Sun . . . . . 5 times
2. Relaxation . . . . . .
3. Head Stand (Group 1). . . . . 1 minute
4. Relaxation . . . . . .
5. Plough Asana (Group 2) . . . . 1 minute
6. Relaxation . . . . . .
7. Bow Asana (Group 4) . . . . . 15 seconds (5 times)
8. Relaxation . . . . . .
9. Salute to the Sun . . . . . 5 times
10. Breath-control . . . . . . 5 minutes

153

Third Stage

1. Salute to the Sun . . . . . 10 times
2. Relaxation . . . .
3. Head Stand (Group 1). . . . . 1 minute
4. Relaxation . . . .
5. Pincers Asana (Group 9) . . . . 4 times
6. Complete Asana (Group 2) . . . . 1 minute
7. Relaxation . . . .
8. Wheel Asana (Group 3) . . . . 4 times
9. Bow Asana (Group 4) . . . . . 4 times
10. Relaxation . . . .
11. Diamond Asana (Group 8) . . . . 3 minutes
12. Locust Asana (Group 6) . . . . 10 seconds (5 times)
13. Relaxation . . . .
14. Head Stand (Group 1). . . . . 1 minute
15. Relaxation . . . .
16. Breath-control . . . . . . 5 minutes or more
17. Salute to the Sun . . . . . 10 times

It is wise for anyone who wishes to apply this method in a regular way to practise the exercises in the following order:

First Stage, for three months.

Second Stage, for three months.

Third Stage, for six months and then modify the asanas so as to make them more and more difficult.

For preference always start with the Salute to the Sun. Finish in the same way and do a few minutes' breath control. If possible, after every training session, drink a large glass of milk or water and lie down for a few minutes.

In a few months your body will be slim and well-proportioned, your voice will become stronger and deeper, and you will feel younger and full of energy and mental poise.

But always remember that Nature refuses to be rushed. She can only be made to evolve. And that takes time.

Take heart!

SUGGESTIONS FOR FURTHER READING

ALAIN: *Yoga for Perfect Health* (Thorsons).

BERNARD, Theos: *Hatha Yoga* (Rider).

BERNARD, Theos: *Heaven Lies Within Us* (Rider).

BERNARD, Theos: *Philosophical Foundations of India* (Rider).

BRUNTON, Paul: *The Inner Reality* (Rider).

DAY, Harvey: *About Yoga* (Thorsons).

DAY, Harvey: *The Study & Practice of Yoga* (Thorsons).

FRANCIS, P. G.: *Yoga—The Amazing Life Science* (Thorsons).

PRABHAVANANDA, Swami, and ISHERWOOD, Christopher, trs.: *The Song of God Bhagavad-Gita* (Phoenix House).

PRABHAVANANDA, Swami, and ISHERWOOD, Christopher, trs.: *How to Know God* (Allen & Unwin).

RADHAKRISHNAN, S.: *The Bhagavadgita* (Allen & Unwin).

WOOD, Ernest E.: *Practical Yoga* (Rider).

YESUDIAN, Selvarajan, and HAICH, Elisabeth: *Yoga and Health* (Allen & Unwin).

YESUDIAN, Selvarajan, and HAICH, Elisabeth: *Yoga Uniting East and West* (Allen & Unwin).

YOGANANDA, Paramhansa: *Autobiography of a Yogi* (Rider).

GLOSSARY OF SANSKRIT TERMS

ARDHA-CHAKRASANA: Half-wheel asana (Group 27).

ARDHA-VRICHIKASANA: Half-scorpion asana (Group 17).

ASANA: Posture.

ASTHA VAKRASANA: Asana of the eight curves (Group 10).

AUM TAT SAT: Father, Son, Holy Ghost.

BADDHA PADMASANA: Locked lotus asana (Group 28).

BHAKTI YOGA: One of the four different types of Yoga for different temperaments, Bhakti Yoga being for emotional temperaments.

BHEGASANA: Bird asana (Group 21).

BHUJANGASANA: Cobra asana (Group 5).

CHAKRASANA: Wheel asana (Group 3).

DAKSHINA NAULI: Internal strengthening exercise involving isolation of the abdominal muscles on the right side (Group 30).

DHANURASANA: Bow asana (Group 4).

DHRITYASANA: Asana of firmness (Group 3).

EKAPADAHASTASANA: One-legged asana, single-footed asana (Groups 19 and 26).

GARBHASANA: Foetus asana (Group 29).

GOKARNASANA: Gokarna asana (Group 13).

GOMUKHASANA: Cow's-head asana (Group 18).

HALASANA: Plough asana (Group 2).

HASTA-PADASANA: Toe-hold asana (Group 14).

HATHA YOGA: Yoga of physical and mental control.

JANUSIRASANA: Head-and-knees asana (Groups 13 and 21).

JNANA YOGA: One of the four different types of Yoga for different temperaments, Jnana Yoga being for intellectual temperaments.

KAKASANA: Raven asana (Group 10).

KAPODASANA: Bird's-head asana (Group 21).

KARMA YOGA: One of the four different types of Yoga for different temperaments, Karma Yoga being for active temperaments.

KONASANA: Angle asana (Group 9).

KRISHNASANA: Asana of Krishna, an incarnation of God who appeared in India about 1400 B.C.

KRIYAS: Internal cleansing exercises (Group 30).

KUKKUTASANA: Cock asana (Group 29).

KURMASANA: Tortoise asana (Group 14).

LAYA YOGA: One of the three main branches of Raja Yoga (q.v.).

LOLASANA: Balance asana (Group 25).

MADYAMA NAULI: Internal strengthening exercise involving isolation of the abdominal muscles in the centre (Group 30).

MANDUKASANA: Frog asana (Group 8).

MANTRA YOGA: One of the three main branches of Raja Yoga (q.v.).

MATSYASANA: Fish asana (Group 24).

MATSYENDRASANA: Asana of Matsyendra, one of the great Yogis of ancient India (Group 20).

MAYURASANA: Peacock asana (Group 11).

MUDRA: Seal.

NATARAJASANA: Dancing asana (Group 12).

NAULI: Internal strengthening exercise involving isolation of the abdominal muscles (Group 30).

PADANGUSHTASANA: Tiptoe asana (Group 15).

PADASIRSHASANA: A variation of the cobra asana (Group 16).

PADMASANA: Lotus asana (Group 22).

PARBATASANA: Mountain asana (Group 23).

PASCHIMOTTANASANA: Pincers asana (Group 9).

PATANJALI: The traditional founder of Yoga.

PRANA: Breath.

PURNA-DHANURASANA: Complete bow asana (Group 12).

PURNA-SUPTA-VAJRASANA: A variation of the diamond asana (Group 16).

RAJA YOGA: One of the four different types of Yoga for different temperaments, Raja Yoga being for intellectual temperaments.

SALABHASANA: Locust asana (Group 6).

SARVANGASANA: Complete asana (Group 2).

SEDHUBANDHASANA: Bridge asana (Group 2).

SIDHASANA: Disciple asana, adept asana (Groups 8 and 15).

SIRSHASANA: Head stand (Group 1).

SVASTIKASANA: Prosperity asana (Group 15).

SWAMI: Master.

TRIKONASANA: Triangle asana (Group 7).

UDDIYANA BANDHA: Drawing in the abdomen (Group 30).

URDWA-PADMASANA: Inverted lotus asana (Group 23).

URDWA-PASCHIMOTTANASANA: Raised pincers asana (Group 27).

UTTITHA-KURMASANA: Upright tortoise asana (Group 26).

UTTITHA-PADMASANA: Raised lotus asana (Group 25).

VAJRASANA: Diamond asana (Group 8).

VAMANA NAULI: Internal strengthening exercise involving isolation of the abdominal muscles on the left side (Group 30).

VATYANASANA: Half-leg asana (Group 22).

VIPARITA-HALASANA: Inverted plough asana (Group 16).

VIRASANA: Hero asana (Group 15).

VRICHIKASANA: Scorpion asana (Group 17).

VRIKSHASANA: Tree asana (Group 1).

YOGA: One of the six classic philosophical systems of ancient India.

YOGA-MUDRA: Yoga seal (Group 28).

INDEX

Numbers in italics refer to illustration number
Numbers in bold type to page numbers